Natural Remedies

For

Animal First Aid

Mark Gilberd
Homoeopath. Medical Herbalist and Iridologist

Index

Index Of Herbal Actions

Alterative, Analgesic, Antibiotic, Anti Catarrhal, Anti Emetic, Anti-Fungal, Anti Inflammatory, Anti Lithic, Anti-Microbial, Anti-Oxidant, Anti Rheumatic, Anti-Tumor, Anti Spasmodic, Anti-viral, Anthelmintic,

Aperient, Astringent, Bitter, Carminative, Cardio active, Circulatory Tonic, Cholagogue, Demulcent, Diaphoretic, Diuretic, Emmenagogue, Emollient, Expectorant, Febrifuge, Galactagogue, Hypotensive, Hypertensive, Hepatic, Hormone Balancers, Immune Booster, Laxative, Nervine, Parasiticide, Pectoral, Rubefacient, Sialagogue, Stimulant, Sedative, Tonic, Urinary Antiseptics, Vermifuge, Vulnerary.

Herbal Supplement
Important Please Read
Introduction To Herbal Medicine
Making Herbal Formulas
How To Make Herbal Tinctures
Hoe To Make Herbal Infusions
How To Make Decoctions
How To Make Poultices
Dosage for Forms Of Herbal Medicine

Herbal
Agrimony, Alfalfa, Angelica, Aniseed, Arnica, Astragalus, Barberry, Bear Berry, Black Cohosh, Blue Flag, Boswella, Broom, Burdock, Buchu, Cayenne, Calendula, Cat Mint, Cats Claw, Celery Seed, Centaury, Chamomile, Chaparral, Chaste Tree, Chickweed, Cleavers, Coltsfoot, Comfrey, Corn Silk, Cranesbill, Cranberry, Dandelion, Devils Claw, Dong Quai, Echinacea, Elecampane, Elder, Eyebright, Fennel, Fenugreek, Feverfew, Figwort, Fumitory,

Garlic, Guaiacum, Gentian, Ginger, Gingko Biloba, Ginseng Panax, Ginseng Siberian, Goldenrod, Gravel Root, Grindelia, Hawthorn, Hops, Horehound, Horse Chestnut, Horseradish, Horsetail, Hypericum, Hyssop, Juniper, Kelp, Ladys Mantle, Lemon Balm, Licorice, Lime Blossom, Marshmallow, Meadowsweet, Mistletoe, Milk Thistle, Motherwort, Mullein, Myrrh, Nasturtium, Neem, Nettles, Oats, Parsley, Passion Flower, PauD'arco, Pennyroyal, Plantain, Peppermint, Poke Root, Raspberry, Red Clover Reshi, Rose Hips, Rosemary, Rue Sage, Sarsaparilla, Shitake, Slippery Elm Bark, Shepherds Purse, Skullcap, St Johns Wort, Sweet Violets, Senna Pods, Tansy, Tea Tree Oil, Thyme, Valerian, Vervain, Wild Yam, Willow Bark, Witch Hazel, Withania Wood Betony, Wormwood, Yarrow, Yellow Dock. Yucca

Homoeopathic Suppplement
Symptoms Guide
Disease Nosodes
How to Make a Nosode In A Hurry

Materia Medica
Aconite, Allium Cepa, Ant Tart, Apis, Arnica, Arsenic Album, Belladonna, Bellis Perinnis, Bryonia, Calendula, Cantharis, Carbo Vegetabilis, Causticum, Euphrasia, Hypericum, Ipecac, Kali Bich, Kali Carb, Lachesis, Ledum, Lycopodium, Nat Sulf, Nux Vom, Phosphorus, Pulsatilla, Rhus Tox, Ruta, Silica,

Staphysagria, Symphytum, Tarantula Cuba, Urtica Urens.

The Safest Essential Oils For Animal Use

Foreword

Natural Remedies For Cats, Dogs and Horses don't have a full herbal of animal herbs mainly for safety reasons while all the other animal books do. For those who have the other books the main interest in this one would be The Index To Herbal Actions which references all the herbs in the Herbal. In the other books you had an Actions Reference at the end of each chapter for each of the body systems. Another important part not in any of the other books is How To Make Disease Nosodes In A Hurry in the Homoeopathic Section. This booklet is set out in four main sections the first being a general First Aid for most animals which is very general as there are a lot of different types of animals but this mainly tries to cover our farm animals and pets. This book is meant to be used mainly as a reference book for some of my other books. Always refer to the herbal actions you require as the actions will put you on to the needed herbs. The second part of the book goes into the herbs that are and have been traditionally used on animals. There are over a hundred different herbs that are mentioned and they would cover most of the conditions known. Information on the actions and uses of these herbs are given along with the dose for a human. The reason I did this is because it makes it easy for you to work out the dose for an animal using the chart in the Herbal Section. The next section is the most important of them all for this gives you a list of actions and the herbs that are best at these actions. For an example we will use a dog with say an infected abscess which is very inflamed and painful. The actions we would want here would be anti-inflammatory; we know that abscesses are caused by bacteria so another action we would want would be anti-bacterial. The dog has been getting this problem on and off for a year so there must be some underlying problem so to treat this we shall choose some Alteratives to clean out the whole system. Now that we know what actions we need eg - Alterative, anti-inflammatory and anti-bacterial we can start looking at the herbs under these listings and read up about them to see which ones suit our case best. This booklet now opens a whole new world to you and puts your animals health care into your own hands but always remember it is better to take the best from all the health providers. The next section is a Homeopathic Materia Medica which gives you information on the homeopathic remedies that are commonly used in First Aid along with some of the commonly used remedies. Most of the first aid remedies are used in the 6C potency which makes them a very broad based remedy. You only use the higher potencies when you have a close match between the symptoms of the patient and the actions of the remedy. You could give these gentle potencies with an Herbal Formula if you wished. I have also added the Essential Oil Section at the end so you have an all in on reference book of animal remedies.

Animal Natural Remedy Books
Natural Remedies For Cat Health
Natural Remedies For Dog Health
Natural Remedies For Goat Health
Natural Remedies For Sheep Health
Natural Remedies For Pig Health
Natural Remedies For Cow Health
Natural Remedies For Horse Health
Natural Remedies For Poultry Health

Mark Gilberd, Homoeopath, Iridologist, Medical Herbalist
Accredited With The Australian Traditional Medicine Society

First Aid Remedies

Always think of safety first, know in your mind what you are going to do and how you are going to do it. Have the right safety gear to protect yourself from bites and kicks. Always remember that injured animals can be dangerous and will lash out if you hurt them more so plan your work carefully.

We will be using both Herbal and Homoeopathic treatment, taking the best from both of them as and when we need it. Out main remedies are going to be Calendula and Hypericum (Saint John's Wort) used in tincture form which we will make lotions to be applied to the wounds.

One of the best ways to learn Homoeopathy and prove to yourself its worth is by getting to know and using some of the main First Aid Remedies. We won't go into too much detail as Homoeopathy can be a Vast and complex form of medicine. Most of the controversy is caused by the use of Potencies. For First Aid we will most of the time use the low potencies usually from 6C to 30C. An example is Arnica 6C is a Low potency while Arnica 30C is the highest of the low potencies. Paradoxically the higher the potency the stronger the action, this is the opposite of Allopathic Medicine which is our normal modern medicine. Low potencies of about 6C can be given every half hour while 30C can be 4 to 5 hourly or sometimes daily. With Homoeopathy you try to match the intensity of the symptom to the potency eg the more intense the pain the higher the potency.

Homoeopathy means literally Same Disease. The law of Homoeopathy is Let Likes Cure Likes. This is important, it is likes cure likes not vaguely similar. If it is only vaguely similar use a low potency eg 6C, if you are sure it's a close match use 30C.

If you want to learn more about Homoeopathic First Aid one of the best books about the subject was written by Dr Dorothy Shepherd (The Magic Of The Minimum Dose) who used most of the remedies below during the Nazi Blitz of London and gives you good examples from her patients.

Our Two Main Wound Herbs
Calendula

Medicinal Actions - Anti-inflammatory, astringent, vulnerary, anti-fungal, germicide, demulcent.

Part Used - The Flowers

Used For.-. Minor skin problems, cuts, abrasions, rashes, spots, acne, sore nipples Slow healing wounds, skin ulcers and to improve post-operative healing Fungal skin infections such as thrush, athletes foot and ring worm. Used to stop bleeding, heal bruises and sprains, skin ulcers, minor burns and scolds, healing, soothing, anti-microbial. As a douche or bath to treat vaginal thrush, Gargle for sore throat and tonsillitis It can be applied as a lotion, ointment, wash, gargle, compress, poultice, bath and douche as required. Use as a lotion (1 to 20) to clean wounds, one of our main germicides for wounds and if Hypericum is added to the lotion you may prevent tetanus as well

Caution - Calendula closes wounds rapidly so make sure they are very clean and no foreign bodies remain.

How To Use – For very serious wound bleeding medicate cloth with tincture and apply with pressure to the area till bleeding stops. Use as a Lotion one part tincture to twenty parts water to wash out wounds or medicate affected area, make at 1 to 10 for bleeding or fungal infections. Use a teaspoon of tincture to medicate a small jar of cream then stir rapidly for 5 minutes or less if it mixes in fast, usually they don't. I usually get a cheap Vitamin E cream from one of the big cheap wholesalers and medicate the cream with Calendula. Use Tincture for medicating creams.

History - The common name for Calendula officinalis is Marigold and it is also known as pot or garden marigold or Mary's Gold. The Latin name is derived from the Latin term calends, which became our English word for calendar, and describes its nature to flower in almost every month of the year. The petals were used by the Romans as a substitute for saffron. The flower petals of calendula or pot marigold, have been used for medicinal purposes since at least the 12th century. Calendula is native to the Mediterranean. Europeans have long used the orange petals of Calendula to color butter and cheese. The use of Marigold as a medicinal plant has been recorded in traditional herbal literature for hundreds of years. Culpepper's Complete Herbal (1653) describes marigolds as 'being so plentiful in every garden, and so well known that they need no description'. Calendula was eaten widely at this time which is where it gets its name, pot marigold i.e. for the cooking pot. Both Culpepper describes its use as a soothing treatment for skin inflammation, swelling, infections, ulcers and varicose veins. It was also found to be beneficial against smallpox and measles to reduce fever and bring out the spots and hence healing.

Herbal Actions of Calendula

Germicide - Calendula is a strong antiseptic, due to it wide variety of chemical constituents, including **carotenoids** which speed up wound healing and strengthens cells. Along with fighting bacteria in topical preparations, Calendula also fights viruses and fungi, particularly those on the skin and nails. Preventing infections means having a healthy immune system, and here the ability of Calendula to cleanse the lymphatic system comes into play. A sluggish immune system is nearly always characterized by poor lymphatic function. So by improving the health of the lymphatic system, Calendula indirectly supports healthy immunity

Anti-inflammatory - Where-ever there is skin irritation and redness, an anti-inflammatory action is needed to help the skin recover. With Calendula also being a Germicide it also takes out the cause of the inflammation which is usually infection. Here the **triterpene alcohols** in calendula exert their powerful inflammation reducing effects. They contribute to the plants overall ability to heal wounds such as burns, cuts and grazes as effectively or more effectively than conventional steroidal applications.

Astringent - The most important use of the astringents in First Aid is to stop the bleeding and they do this by causing the arterioles and arteries to spasm at the cut end. Calendula is well known for stopping bleeding especially in the hard to stop areas such as the palms of hands where in the serious cases tinctures can be used on cloth and put in the palm and the patient made to make a fist. Calendulas astringent action can be used to improve blood vessel tone and tighten up skin cells. The plant also contains **flavonoids** which improve circulation by boosting the health of capillaries.

Demulcent - The soothing properties of Calendula are due to many of its chemical constituents, in particular the **triterpene saponins** and **mucilage**. Both of these substances provide a demulcent' healing effect on external skin surfaces. Another significant component of Calendula is the **essential oil** which is used in many skin formulations and is aromatic.

Hypericum
(St Johns Wort)

Medicinal Actions - Anti-inflammatory, astringent, anti-viral, anti-spasmodic, nervine, vulnerary, antibacterial.

Part Used - Aerial parts

Uses – For First Aid we are concentrating on external use only. Used for wounds with pains that shoot along the nerves, in nerve rich areas such as the fingers, lips, tail bone and toes. As a lotion it will speed the healing of wounds and bruises and is used where there is nerve damage and the possibility of tetanus. The main remedy for puncture wounds. Good for, varicose veins especially the painful kind and mild burns. Patients recovering from surgery where the nerves have been damaged often recover faster with Hypericum. For inflamed joints and rheumatic pain, painful abscesses, bad insect stings, damaged nerves from impact injuries, sprains and ulcers. Eases the pain in conditions such as lumbago, sciatica and Shingles where a cream can be used on the sore and the oil applied along the affected nerve path. As a lotion it is commonly mixed with Calendula, Homoeopaths call this lotion Hypercal.

How To Use - Use as a Lotion one part tincture to twenty parts water to wash out wounds or medicate affected area, make at 1 to 10 for painful and dirty wounds. Mix with Calendula in large painful bleeding wounds with a chance of tetanus. Use Tincture for medicating creams.

History

St. John's Wort has enjoyed a reputation as a wound healer since the fifth century BC. Dioscorides, Paul of Aegina, Pliny, and Galen all referred to the plant, which is said to relieve excessive pain, remove the effects of shock, and have a tonic effect on the mind and body. The name St. John probably refers to John the Baptist, whom tradition said was born on the summer solstice. It was claimed that the red spots visible on the underside of some of the herb's leaves symbolized the blood of St. John, who was beheaded by Herod. In **1907 Ellingwood** a famous Herbalist of the time listed the uses as for muscular bruises, deep soreness, painful parts, a sensation of throbbing in the body without fever. Burning pain, or deep soreness of the spine upon pressure, spinal irritation, and circumscribed areas of intense soreness over the spinal cord or ganglia. Concussional shock or injury to the spine, lacerated or punctured wounds in any location, accompanied with great pain. In the times of horse and carriages Homoeopaths were using it on horses to prevent tetanus after injuries to the hoofs mainly from puncture wounds there from nails or similar objects as these wound on the hoof were prone to tetanus. Hypericum has been one of the main Homoeopathic First Aid Remedies for hundreds of years used by itself or mixed with Calendula in a solution called HYPERCAL. After the 1930's it faded from popularity, but was used by the Russians in WW2 as a replacement for morphine in Lotion and Potencies

Hypercal

Hypercal is a 50 50 mixture of Hypericum and Calendula Tinctures. This is a combination of two of the best wound healing herbs mixed together. Calendula is more for dealing with the blood vessels and bleeding along with the rapid closure of the wound so care must be taken to ensure the wound is clean and no foreign bodies are there to be sealed in. Hypericums work is more on the damaged nerves and pain as well as infections in and of the nervous system especially those caused by deep and painful puncture wounds which could harbor tetanus if not properly cleaned and dealt with. By using these two herbs together you are doubling their main actions of anti-inflammatory and astringents with the last action being good for stopping bleeding and also infection. Wounds calling for Hypercal are usually bloody and painful. Works well on long and extensive grazes and cleaning gravel rash and wounds but is mainly called for impact injuries to the lips, fingers or toes. Ideal for closing clean incisions fast and after surgical operations. So the leading symptoms for Hypercal are painful wounds.

Use as a lotion at one part to ten or 1 to 20 depending on your judgment of pain and infection. In emergency bleeding use the tincture as this will spasm the arterioles but be aware that the high alcohol content will cause pain in its raw state. Use Tincture for medicating creams.

Abscesses - Boils and Carbuncles

These are typically caused by a bacterial infection usually starting in a hair follicle or from a deep infected wound usually from a bite especially in Cats. The first stage is characterized by a painful red swelling after which pus begins to form; this will usually discharge itself in a few days. Do not squeeze as this usually causes internal damage and a spread of the wound and infection.

Herbal Treatment

The easiest and fasted method would be to use Tea Tree Oil as this tends to draw out infections and bring them to a head. Start as soon as possible, the earlier the better and apply frequently. Use more diluted if using frequently especially if you have sensitive pets and think twice about using on Cats as they don't like oils. Hot poultices are very effective at drawing the core out of boils so here we shall use a hot poultice of Slippery Elm (half a tea spoon full) with about 4 drops of Castor Oil which is also good at drawing out unwanted matter and mix this with a bit of boiling water to form a hot paste. Alternative poultices are Linseed or Fenugreek, these need to be ground and boiled first before being applied. Apply to the area and leave on for 20 minutes and repeat several times till suppuration occurs.

After suppuration you can mix together a bit of Calendula and Hypericum in cream or lotion form and apply them to the area. These two herbs working together will speed up the healing time, disinfect and reduce or prevent scaring. If you think it was caused from a puncture wound think more of Hypericum as this was the old treatment for tetanus.

For internal treatment for boils that keep on reoccurring think of the herbs Echinacea and Burdock as these are both blood cleansers that will start to work on the causes of the problem and help to prevent more.

Homoeopathic Treatment

A boil is an infected, reddened, swollen area of the skin usually in a hair follicle or some other pit in the skin. Boils can be very painful while they develop until they come to a head and burst.

Hypericum Lotion - Make at a strength of 1 to 25 parts water, soak a compress and apply reasonably wet to the affected area. Take Tarantula at the time.

Hepar Sulph 6C - To ripen a slow forming boil or abscess.

Silica 6C - For more advanced boils to encourage them to discharge, for foul smelling discharges or incomplete discharges.

Arnica 6C - For crops of boils with a bluish area around them.

Tarantula Cubenis 6C - For painful hard feeling boils that develop rapidly after a slow start where the skin turns red blue or purple. Give this remedy 3 or 4 times daily along with a Hypericum Lotion compress taped over the area.

Bites and Stings

I will cover here just bites from animals and bee and wasp stings. Snakes spiders and jellyfish stings require prompt medical attention. With snake and spider bites apply a pressure bandage to the area and keep the limb still and transport or call the vet. Give Homoeopathic Ledum immediately and try to identify the snake or spider to make it easier for the vet. (You can give Rescue Remedy).

Animal bites can be treated the same as wounds as they are usually a mixture of puncture, bruising and maybe scratches, treat shock with Rescue Remedy or give Homoeopathic Ledum immediately as this is the specific for puncture wounds. Treat with lots of Calendula Lotion so as to prevent infection which is common after animal bites especially from cats. If there is a lot of pain add Hypericum to the lotion. Always add the Hypericum to Calendula in bites and deep puncture wounds as Hypericum was the old remedy for preventing tetanus.

Herbal Treatment

For insect bites and stings Rescue Remedy taken internally and applied to the sting can bring relief especially in kittens and pups. Witch hazel cream is good for insect bites and stings.

Wasp stings and Ant bites - apply vinegar or lemon juice

Bee stings - Dab on bicarbonate of soda mixed with water. This can also bring relief to sand fly and sometimes mosquito bites as well. Baking Soda works in two ways, firstly it buffers the acid and then the sodium part draws the poison out. On all stings ice can reduce pain and swelling. Aloe vera may sometimes help.

Homoeopathic Treatment

Always follow the normal first aid procedures especially from bites from venomous creatures. After a bite or a sting from an animal or insect take one dose of **Ledum 6C** immediately. If you get no relief try one of the following.

Apis 6C - If the injury swells, burns, stings and looks very red, angry and puffy with swelling, worse for warmth , better for cold applications. This remedy is made from the bee and should always be considered for bee stings.

Arnica 6C - Shock, bruising like pain, soreness and does not want area touched.

Cantharis 6C - Violent burning and smarting pain, blisters may develop.

Staphysagria 6C - Large bites that itch violently with smarting, stinging pain.

Bruises and Suspected Bruises

Arnica is the main remedy that is used for bruising mainly as a lotion or a cream but it must not be used where the skin is broken. If used on broken skin it will cause a bad reaction. Arnica is good for the bruised like pains in limbs and joints which have been over used or sprained as well as your everyday type of bruises. For accidents especially impact injuries on limbs use ice or cold water tap and leave it there till you think it nearly feels numb with the cold, this if done fast enough save the victim from a lot of pain and damage.

Herbal Treatment

For bruises where there are open wounds such as cuts and grazes use Witch hazel and Calendula together in a lotion and later you could mix the creams together and apply as healing resumes. For your normal everyday bruises rub Arnica cream gently on the area. (never rub hard as you could put a clot into the blood stream). If a nerve rich area such as the elbow is bruised add Hypericum to the lotion.

For internal treatment give a Vitamin C powder with

hesperidin, rutin and the bioflavonoids as this will help to repair the damaged capillaries. If the patient bruises easily consider giving this powder regularly as they may be deficient.

Homoeopathic Treatment

The black and blue appearance of a bruise are caused from blood vessels that have ruptured under the skin as a result of trauma, as the blood from the broken vessels is slowly absorbed the color becomes paler then red or yellow though this can be hard to see under the fur and the color doesn't come out immediately.

Arnica 6C - For bruised soft tissues, muscles and connective tissue. Rapidly aids in the absorption of effused blood. The swelling which usually accompany bruising reduces fairly quickly but if there is little reaction use Ledum 6C. Arnica cream can be used on the external area of the wound.

Caution - Arnica lotion or cream must not be used on or near broken skin only use Calendula or Hypericm cream on wounds.

Ledum 6C - Helps in blood reabsorbing, may be needed if swelling remains after taking Arnica. Affected parts are cold and worse for warmth.

Hypericum 6C - For bruised nerves, use where there is sharp shooting pains in punctured or penetrating wounds, for bruises of nerve rich areas such as the fingers, tail bone, lips and nose. Hypercal cream can be applied to the site externally.

Ruta 6C - Bruises of the bone or the bone covering

the periosteum, good for shin bone injuries.

Note - Hypercal cream can be used externally on bruises where the skin is broken as Arnica cream or lotion cannot be used on broken skin.

Bleeding

The main rule for bleeding is to apply pressure to the wound so as to stop the bleeding. For a normal type of slow blood flow from a wound that is persistent Calendula tincture applied with pressure on a pad will usually stop the bleeding, make sure you hold it there for a few minutes.

For the more scary type of bleeding Witch hazel tincture can be used on a pad and applied with pressure to the wound as this herb is much more astringent then Calendula, this extra astringency should cause the ends of the blood vessels to spasm and close off the injured vessels.

Herbal Treatment

Calendula for slow bleeding wounds.

Witch hazel for the fast bleeding wounds.

I would be inclined here to mix the tincture half water half tincture as this would still work and be less painful as the alcohol in the tincture is much more reduced.

See also Cuts and Wounds and consider using Hypercal (Hypericum and Calendula mixed together)

Homoeopathic Treatment

Use normal first aid procedures, apply pressure to the wound, if there is a lot of blood loss seek medical help and be on the lookout for shock.

Arnica 6C - For bleeding after injury, helps with the shock and bruising.

Bone Injuries and Fractures

Follow normal first aid procedures, if the bone is obviously broken you have to decide on your response taking into consideration your personal safety. If you do have to move the patient make sure the injured limb is supported or a sharp piece of bone may cut an internal artery. Fast strong splints can be made from plastic plumbing pipe cut down to size then split through the center long ways. Bandages can then be used to tie the splint into place though you may find electrical insulation tape is a fast and easy way to go especially on the smaller animal or on birds where we sometimes use a drink straw as a splint. Most bone injuries need x-rays to determine the extent of the damage. Use Arnica 6C or higher for the shock and pain or Rescue Remedy.

Herbal Treatment

The main remedy here is Comfrey or to use its old fashioned name knitbone. This is good to use on the injured area when the cast is removed as it will help to strengthen the mend. For areas that cannot have casts on or for fine fractures Comfrey is ideal and will speed up the healing process.

Comfrey has a chemical in it that speeds up cell division it is also astringent and mucilage which gives it soothing and protecting qualities and has been used for hundreds of years in the healing of bones and wounds. Some people grow this herb and then turn it into liquid manure as it is one of the most mineral rich herbs around. Apply cream to affected area regularly, if you grow comfrey in your garden you can make a poultice out of the leaves and apply it to the affected area.

Homoeopathic Treatment

Arnica 6C - Can be given straight away for the shock and will help ease the pain from the bruising and swelling.

Ledum 6C - Take after Arnica 4 hourly or 3 times a day to assist in the absorption of the extravasation of blood after a fracture so as to reduce the swelling which may take up to 3 to 4 days. (Helps to absorb the internal bleeding after a fracture)

After the bones have been set properly use these two remedies

Calc Phos 6X - Helps in nutrition especially of the bones and promotes the knitting together of the bones. Helps fractures heal much faster. Can be used in alternation with Symphytum 6C.

Symphytum 6C - More commonly known as Comfrey or knitbone or bone set. The name says it all. Promotes fast healing of bones, use with Calc Phos 6X. Take both 3 times daily till recovered.

Burns

Get all burns under cold water immediately; always

remember that burns keep on burning inwards for about 15 seconds after the heat source is removed. On first degree burns the skin becomes red only. 2nd degree the burn begins to destroy living tissue, blisters develop, 3rd degree the burns are deep and involve all layers of the skin, these are life threatening depending on the size of the area mainly through the loss of fluids and the risk of infections.

Herbal Treatment

For minor burns and scolds Aloe Vera gel straight from the plants leaf can give quick relief and speed up the healing. In herbalism we use astringents for burns (with the exception being for burns that cover a very large area) as the tannins in the herbs will seal and protect the burned surface. Deep burns always require prompt medical attention.

Treatment

Aloe Vera - Apply to burn straight from the plant.

Witch Hazel - Use as a lotion at about 1 to 20 strength and apply to the burn, this herb is a strong astringent and should seal and protect the surface.

Once the healing has begun you can continue applying Aloe era especially if there is still pain. Another good herb for the pain is Hypericum which you could apply as a lotion. Calendula cream can also be applied to the healing edges of the wound.

Homoeopathic Treatment

Calendula Cream - Use this on the edges of the burn as the burn heals.

Causticum 6C to 30C - For 2nd degree burns

taken as needed for the pain with Hypericum lotion used externally on the burn and calendula cream on the edges.

Cantharis 6C to 30C - For 3rd degree burns taken as needed. This time wait for the healing to begin before using Hypericum and calendula as mentioned with Causticum.

Hypericum 6C to 30C - To be used as a lotion 20 drops of tincture to 1 cup of water. (soothes the pain).

Urtica Urens 6C to 30C - For first degree burns taken as needed internally for the pain with Hypericum lotion used externally.

Cuts and Wounds

The first consideration is to stop the bleeding, rule out any deeper internal damage and clean and disinfect the wound. To stop the bleeding refer to the bleeding section. Calendula is one of the main lotions used for cleaning wounds as it is gentle, soothing, astringent, healing and anti-microbial so it kills the germs as well. Calendula has a tendency of sometimes welding the skin together (handy for closing knife cuts) this is more noticeable on wounds with clean cut edges. Because of this tendency it is very important to make sure that all wounds are very clean and no dirt remains inside. Now we will introduce you to Hypericum (St Johns Wort) I use Hypericum lotion on wounds that are in very nerve rich areas, a good example is crush injuries to the finger as we all know how painful and sensitive a wound is to this area. So for animals it's the hoof areas where we also need it for its tetanus prevention, lips and nose area or any area that you judge is extra nervy and twitchy. As well as being used for nerve damage Hypericm is also astringent so it will help in stopping the bleeding and its anti-inflammatory action should help to reduce the swelling. I usually get a separate bottle and fill it up with half Hypericum and half Calendula tincture and call this bottle Hypercal. I use this bottle for making my lotions for wounds on nervy areas or large graze areas as these are also highly sensitive and raw. Consider also that these are both astringents so our power to stop bleeding has been increased.

Tea Tree Oil is good for small wounds and has a strong antibacterial action but can sometimes hurt in open wounds. The oil is good where there is infection as it draws pus to a head, but don't use on cats and birds as they don't like the Essential Oils. If you are going to try to get away without stitches try to immobilize the area for a couple of days so you don't accidentally rip the wound open again and use plenty of Calendula to close the wound and confine the animal to the shed or barn.

Herbal Treatment

1. Deal with bleeding and clean wound under running tap water if possible.
2. Do the final cleaning with Calendula or Hypercal lotion mixed 1 to 20 parts water.
3. Cover and protect the wound if you think it is

necessary, especially if lots of flies and irritating insects are about.

4. When wound is dry and healing (if weeping use Hypercal lotion) you can use Calendula cream with maybe Comfrey cream as well for scar prevention or if the wound is healing slowly. You can also medicate a little bit of Calendula cream with Hypericum to make a Hypercal cream for a healing wound giving off nervy pain.

Homoeopathic Treatment

Use normal first aid techniques, control bleeding etc. When you have everything under control and are ready to see to the wound the best way to start is usually to clean the area with water running from a tap washing everything away from the wound. Calendula lotion is our main treatment for wounds as it is gentle, encourages healing, stops bleeding and no germs can survive in its presence. Use plenty of lotion on the wound and in deep ones let it get into all the cavities. Calendula can make wounds close up very fast especially if they have clean sharp edges so great care must be taken to ensure the wound is clean. Calendula is a great help to old and infected wounds and can usually turn the condition around in a few days. (See Tea Tree oil)

Hypericum is the next most well used lotion, its main calling is for wounds of the very nervy parts of the body such as the fingers, tail bone, lips or for any part that really hurts and is nervy. One of the leading symptoms for Hypericum is shooting pains along the nerve pathways from the injured area. Hypericum is good for infections and septic conditions in nervy areas and I would use it with Calendula for any infection in a wound especially deep wounds. In the past Hypericum was used to prevent Tetanus in deep puncture wounds especially from rusty metal objects. Remember infections are trying to get the rubbish out of the body so when they begin to discharge do not try to stop the discharge let the body get rid of its rubbish.

Hypercal - Which is a half and half mixture of Hypericum and Calendula tinctures, you can use this to make lotions when you want the effects of both Calendula and Hypericum together. An example would be an infected crushed finger.

Creams - Calendula and Hypericum creams can be used when the healing begins and are applied for the same reasons as the lotions but always remember the lotion gets in better and deeper especially if you are using gravity to help. Creams are more for the latter stages of healing.

Arnica 6C - For shock, bruised sore pain of the wound, doesn't like effected area being touched.

Ledum 6C - Used for puncture wounds, prevents tetanus.

Puncture Wounds

Splinters and accidents from stepping on pins, rusty nails, barbed wire or from tools can be dealt with very effectively with homoeopathic remedies.

Arnica 6C - Can help bring splinters to the surface

and deal with any shock.

Hypericum 6C - Intense pain shoots up from injured parts especially from those in nerve rich areas, if given immediately with the lotion it can prevent tetanus from developing but it is always best to get a booster shot.

Ledum 6C - This remedy also helps to prevent tetanus and can be used for the same injuries as Hypericum but with Ledum the part feels cold and is relieved by cold, there is puffiness and a pale mottled appearance.

Hypercal Lotion - Externally use a lotion of Hypercal making sure plenty gets inside the wound.

After Surgery

Homoeopathic remedies used before and immediately after surgery will speed up the healing process considerably. Not only does this get you over the problem sooner but it also helps in the prevention of post-operative complications such as hemorrhage, inflammation, and infection. Will also help with the internal healing and bruising.

Aconite 6C - Great fear and anguish with restlessness. Possible fear of death, great suddenness of symptoms. This is a good one to think of before surgery.

Arnica 6C - Bruised sore pain with fear of being touched. Take this immediately before and straight after a operation.

Bellis Perennis 6C - Follows after and is similar to

Arnica but is used for the deeper internal bruising while Arnica is more external. Good for trauma and wounds of the pelvic and abdominal organs.

Hypericum 6C - For damage to tissue rich in nerves or the nerves themselves, pains shoot along nerve pathways.

Staphysagria 6C - Stinging, cutting, smarting pains after surgery, good for knife cut like wounds. This remedy has strong mental symptoms of Feels as if the body has been invaded, or a sense of humiliation after a physical exam, resentment and anger to medical staff may be present.

Calendula Lotion - This is our main lotion and cream used for wounds. Apply the lotion to the wound and surrounding area as Calendula is very soothing and healing. Latter when the wound is healing Calendula cream can be used.

Hypercal Lotion - Is a mixture of Calendula and Hypericum tinctures that are used as a lotion. The Calendula is used for its healing, anti-microbial, anti-hemorrhagic and soothing properties while the Hypericum is used for the nervy type of pain from the wounds in nerve rich areas.

The lotion is mixed at a strength of 1 to 20 parts water or stronger if needed.

Diarrhea

Diarrhea is a natural bodily process that is used to rid the body of toxins, infections or irritants of any kind so unless it continues for too long it should not be suppressed. Lots of fluids should be taken and in some cases it may be wise to stay off food for 24 hours. Always try to find the cause; it may be from stress, viruses, bacterial infection or overly rich foods or concentrates.

Herbal Treatment

It is important to find out the cause for the best cure is to always remove the cause if you can. Diarrhea is usually treated with astringents usually the milder ones as the very strong ones may upset a sensitive tummy. Some examples are Meadowsweet, Agrimony and Slippery Elm. Going to a more extreme case we shall use for example sheep with black scour which kills off many hill sheep in England. The cause of this is from overeating of rank or very sodden or over rich green food or poisonous plants etc. If treated immediately it is not difficult to cure but if neglected death can occur especially in lambs. Treatment begins with a laxative drench to sweep out the putrid matter from the intestines, a quick and effective drench is one to two ounces of Epsom Salts dissolved in half a pint brew of Dill seeds (one hand full) boiled for 5 minutes in one pint of water or give senna pods. Fast the sheep for 24 hours following the drench and give garlic for internal disinfecting in the evening. The first feed after the fast could be a thin molasses mixed with slippery elm which is a soothing and mild astringent herb. Other herbs to think of are Chamomile, Peppermint and Witch Hazel.

Note - Emergency Rehydration Liquid (electrolytes)

Homemade Electrolyte Solution

Since death results from dehydration and shock the first goal is to restore the electrolyte balance.

2 tablespoons of salt

1 teaspoon of baking soda

8 tablespoons of honey

1 gallon of water.

Homoeopathic Treatment

Aconite 30C- Diarrhea in the primary stage, at the beginning of acute cases that come on suddenly and violently, when it arises from taking cold, considerable fever, inflammation of the bowels, can be alternated with Nux Vom. Dose every half hour for 4 doses.

Nux Vom 12X - Discharges slimy and offensive with rumbling noises in the bowels and passing of wind, when there are symptoms of indigestion and when purging is alternated with constipation for example frequent passing of 1 or 2 small feculent balls accompanied by tenesmus. Dose once every 2 hours.

Arsenicum 1M - For watery, slimy, greenish or brownish diarrhea, with or without gripping pains and can smell offensive, great rumbling in the bowels and flatulence, total loss of appetite and a marked prostration of strength, skin and extremities cold great restlessness. Dose every hour for 4 doses.

China 30C - Useful in chronic cases or when caused by hot weather and not of a inflammatory character, painless discharge, loss of appetite and strength. Can be used as a tonic when acute symptoms have passed away, evacuations consist partly of undigested food , can be pain during discharge.

Bryonia 30C- If the disorder has been brought on by a change of temperature especially from hot to cold, by drinking cold water or impure water, faeces are very watery and involuntary passed and may contain undigested food, can be alternating diarrhea and constipation. Dose four times a day.

Mercurius Cor 200C- Frequent discharge of mucous tinged with blood or thin bloody and foetid stools, frequent urging to stool, redness and swollen appearance of the anus, symptoms worse at night. Dose 3 times daily for 3 days.

Colocynthis 6C - Nausea, severe colicky pains, slimy evacuations or mucous tinged with blood, distension of the bowels and pain on pressure, tenesmus, thirst, variable temperature of the body being at one time shivering and soon after very hot. Dose every half hour for 4 doses.

Chamomilla 30C- If there is pain just before a evacuation which can be of a greenish colour with mucous. Dose four times a day

Note - See also Coccidiosis and Enterotoxaemia in the disease section.

Eye Problems

See also conjunctivitis. Again look to your personal safety first as animals may lash out when you are dealing with the eye. Larger animals in the field tend to draw flies to damaged eyes which make the problem worse and life a misery for the animal so consider using a human face or dust mask as an eye patch. Eyebright as you can guess is the main herb for the eye and is used for most eye problems and even for just sore or strained eyes it can be soothing. For a little splinter in the eye or a hard to remove foreign body a few drops of Castor oil can be used for its drawing power as it has a good reputation for removing embedded objects and it will sooth the irritation at the same time. If the eye is irritated and you have suspicion there is something in put a few drops of Castor oil in before and leave overnight and the problem will usually be gone by the morning.

Herbal Treatment

Eyebright lotion at 1 to 20 parts water in an eyebath (always try in a very diluted form first, 2 drops to a eyebath) for sore red eyes or better still as a compress. Castor oil 2 or 3 drops into the eye to draw out foreign bodies and relieve irritation. Best left overnight. Also see Fennel.

Conjunctivitis

The conjunctiva is a delicate membrane which covers the whites of the eyes. This may become inflamed due to irritation, infection or allergic reaction. Try to avoid touching and rubbing the eye as this usually irritates it more and if it is an infection there is a chance that it may spread to the other eye. The herbs to use here are Calendula and Eyebright used as lotions in the strength of 1 to 20 parts water. Eyebright is a very astringent herb so you would use it if the eye was very watery and inflamed while Calendula is soothing and anti-infective. If the eye was watery and infected you could mix both the herbs together for a more effective treatment.

Herbal Treatment

Calendula lotion 1 to 20 in a eyebath (healing and soothing).

Eyebright Lotion 1 to 20 in a eyebath (astringents will help in stopping watering and help with the inflammation).

Homoeopathic Treatment

Here I will cover mainly blows to the eyes and the simple removal of foreign objects and will also give you one of the main eye remedies. For a blow to the eye you can give Arnica 6C or Aconite 6C which has been called the Arnica of the eye, a leading symptom for Aconite 6C is if the eye feels gritty or as if something is in the eye. If pain is felt in the eyeball give Symphytum 6C.

Arnica 6C is more suited for a black eye (see bruising).

After removal of a foreign object from the eye Aconite 6C can be given and if the eye is still sensitive and sore an eye bath of water with 2 drops of Euphrasia (Eye Bright) tincture can be tried.

Arnica 6C - For shock and bruising.

Acconite 6C - For the suddenness of the condition and shock, pain feels like a piece of grit in the eye, eye looks red and inflamed.

Euphrasia Lotion - Conjunctivitis after injury, eyes are hot, burning and watering, soreness, eye strain. 2 drops of tincture into a eye bath full of water gives relief to sore and wind burnt eyes. You can also use Euphrasia 6C internally at the same time.

Symphytum 6C - for blows to the eyeball itself, blunt injury trauma such as a tennis or squash ball.

Nerve Damage

Herbal Treatment

Damage to the nerves can be very painful and make an area very sensitive. Hypericum is the best remedy for damaged nerves, its main leading symptoms are shooting pains from damaged nerves traveling down the nerve pathways. Another thing to consider is that inflammation can put pressure on nerves and crush them especially the nerves of the spine and around joints so it would be wise to look at the anti-inflammatory herbs as well as the nervines listed in the Herbal Actions section of the book.

Homoeopathic Treatment

Hypericum 30 or 200C - Use for any injury involving nerve damage especially pain in the feet.

Arnica 200C - Used for blows , prevents bruising and stops bleeding.

Ringworm

Ringworm is a fungal infection which usually attacks when the immune system is weakened by stress or exhaustion. Fungi thrive in damp, dark and confined places. If you think your immune system is run down you can take Echinacea, Zinc, and Vitamin C and you might as well take Garlic as this has an anti-fungal action. Externally treatment can be a lotion of Calendula 1 to 5 strength for cleaning the area and around it. Stronger anti fungals may be necessary as this can sometimes be a very stubborn condition to get rid of. Garlic is a stronger anti-fungal and you can use this externally (break open a Garlic oil capsule) and internally at the same time. Other herbs to consider are Burdock, Elder, Myrrh and Rue.

Herbal Treatment

Raise immunity if needed refer to influenza for the method.

Calendula lotion 1 to 5 strength on and around the affected area.

Tea tree oil - strong anti-fungal dab on to the affected area neat.

Garlic externally on effected area and latter if problem is not resolving take internally. Another old remedy to consider is raw lemon juice applied twice daily.

Homoeopathic Remedies

Bacillinum 200C - 2 doses at two week intervals with sepia 6C.

Tellurium 30C - Twice a day for one week especially when lesions tend to be equally distributed on either side of the body.

Chrysarobinum 6C - 3 times a day for 5 days, when the disease has progressed to the crusty stage.

Note - Animals that are susceptible to ringworm are usually deficient in copper. Give a Kelp Supplement or seaweed meal.

Shock

As you would of noticed by now Arnica is our main remedy for shock with Aconite being a very good second remedy if the symptoms match. I have added Rescue Remedy which is not a true homoeopathic remedy but is a close relative and can be used for any type of shock physical or emotional. Emotionally it will relieve that uptight feeling or apprehension before a certain event. Rescue Remedy is a mixture of five Bach Flower Remedies and has been used since the late 1930s so it has been well proved. I have found Rescue Remedy very effective on the young especially kittens and puppies. Don't forget to follow all your normal first aid procedures and keep the patient warm.

Homoeopathic Remedies

Aconite 30C - Severe shock with great fear and

restlessness use first in high potency.

Arnica 30C - Reduces shock and hemorrhage and helps relieve the pain.

Rescue Remedy - For physical and emotional shock in any circumstances.

Sprains and Strains

Severe sprains usually need a supporting bandage and a medical checkup to see if there has been any other damage. A lot of damage and trauma can be prevented if the injured area was put under cold water or ice immediately after the injury the quicker the less the damage. For a bad sprain I would use lots of Arnica cream to start with and at night apply Arnica and Comfrey mixed creams along with a support bandage for the area so as to keep the cream there and also for the extra heat to the area that would create. If you grow Comfrey in your garden then you could put on a Comfrey poultice at night. Ginger is another herb that could be used in a poultice at night. A very fast method of treating strains and sprains is with Glucosamine, Chondroitin and MSM in the powdered form, you should be able to find this at most chemists. Glucosamine is an anti-inflammatory while the chondroitin helps rebuild cartilage and heal joints and attachments. You use this in the powdered form dissolved in water as it is rapidly absorbed by the intestine and enters the blood which takes it to the injury. A lot of athletes and horses use this frequently during the day along with the hot and cold treatment to force heal their injuries so they can compete again as soon as possible. Three times a day is good enough for the rest of us.

Herbal Treatment

Cold water or ice immediately.
Arnica cream (do not apply on open wounds).
Comfrey Cream mixed with Arnica cream overnight.
Ginger poultice overnight.

Homoeopathic Treatment

Joint problems due to twisting, wrenching or over use. A sprain is damaged tendons or ligaments while a strain happens when the connecting tissues around a joint are over stretched. Use your normal first aid procedures and support the joint with supporting bandage and give the appropriate remedies with the first one being Arnica. If there is no sign of improvement in 24 to 36 hours get checked for a fracture.

Arnica 6C - For the shock and bruised sore pains. Arnica cream can also be applied as long as the skin is not broken.

Bellis Perennis 6C - Deeper acting then Arnica, intense soreness of the muscles, where swellings and lumps remain after the injury.

Ledum 6C - Injuries where the swollen part is cold or numb, sometimes looks purple and puffy, feels better for cold applications.

Ruta 6C - If the bones inside or near the joint feel bruised

Tick Bite

Use **Ledum 30C**

Tick Bite Paralysis

Lathyrus Sativus 30C

Tick Paralysis For Dogs

Conium 1M give first.
Gelsemium 10 M to make feel better.
Carbo Veg 1m after if breathing is not good.
Give these remedies half an hour apart. Cynthia Idle.

A Food Supplement For All Animals

In a mixing bowl combine the following ingredients
1 cup of Dolomite Powder
1 and a half cups of Spirulina Powder
1 cup of Kelp Powder
1 cup of Vit C Powder (Super Ascorbate Plus by Hilton Lifestream)
Blend ingredients well and transfer to a air tight container and label.
Cats and Dogs up to 10kg quater to half teas spoon with each meal. 10 to 20kg use 1 level teaspoon, 20 to 40kg use 1 rounded teaspoon,.
Rabbits, Guinea Pigs, Ferrets - quater teaspoon.
Poultry - 1 teaspoon per flock.

Horse - 1 rounded table spoon.

Goats, Sheep, Pigs, Ponies - 1 rounded teaspoon.

Note - For all animals double the dose in late pregnancy and during lactation. Half the dose for infant animals up to 3 months of age.

Introduction To Herbal Medicine

Herbal Medicine has been in use and developed continuously since the beginning of time. It mainly evolved from observations from what plants did and the affects they had on people along with their animals. There is also what they call the Doctrine of Signatures which works like this, that flower really looks like an eye, maybe it helps sore eyes? I'll give it a try as my eyes are so sore and red. You know my eye really feels a lot better now, I think I will call that plant Eye Bright (Euphrasia) and tell my friends all about it especially my Dad who gets sore eyes to. In this way hundreds of plants were identified that have a medical action and no doubt there were also a lot of casualties.

The next great leap in herbal medicine was the Roman Empire of 2000 years ago. The Great Armies of Rome all had their own Medical Corps with Doctors, Battle Surgeons and Orderlies. It was these men who already had the knowledge of the Greeks that started to put together the best medical manuals in the world while at the same time started developing and using medical instruments and tools some of which are still used today. As the Romans conquered the known world more medicines and knowledge were found and assimilated.

The next great leap was modern Chemistry which allowed us to see exactly what herbs were made up of and what parts of the herb causes its medical action. Drug companies have made billions of Dollars from this information as they find the main active ingredient and then make a synthetic version of it, one good example that we all know of is Valium which is the synthetic version of the active ingredient from the herb Valerian. Leaving aside the Drug Companies let's see how Chemistry changed the way that modern herbalists think.

Modern science allows us to now know what Actions our herbs perform on the body so we shall carry on using Valerian as an example and see what Medical Actions Valerian has on the body.

The Actions of Valerian are Sedative, Hypnotic (sleep inducing), Anti Spasmodic (stops twitches, cramps etc), Hypotensive (lowers Blood Pressure) and Carminative (calms and relaxes the tummy). Herbalists call Valerian the Herbal Tranquillizer and if you look at the above you can see why for if you can't sleep and your blood pressures up along with a gurgling tummy and an eye constantly twitching you definitely need to be calmed down.

The modern herbalist is trained to think in actions. There are many reasons for this but the main ones are to stop them from just using a handful of their favorite herbs and to train the mind to work in the method of thinking in actions that are needed. If we start thinking in the actions that are needed for a patient it makes us consider the problem in far more depth than just using our favorite herb and it forces our thinking to be far more holistic by taking in consideration the whole of the patient not just the part or the system we wish to treat.

Let's take a look at thinking in actions. The animal has a cough, but when it coughs it can't stop and the cough sounds a bit like whooping cough. The animal also sounds a little hoarse and the temperature is also elevated. The actions that come into mind for this are expectorant for the cough, anti spasmodics for the whooping quality of the cough and demulcents to sooth the sore throat. These are the obvious actions and we can add many more if we wish such as immune boosters for acute diseases, diaphoretics to reduce the temperature and prevent a fever and the list goes on. Next we look at how Herbal Actions are used in making Herbal Formulas.

Another point to make before we go to the formula making is that Professional Herbalists use Herbs in the form of Tinctures (water and alcohol solutions) as this allows them to mix formulas in any proportions that they like and also allows long term storage without spoiling.

Making Herbal Formulas

You should never have more the 5 Herbs in an herbal formula otherwise you start to lose track of what you are doing and how the formula is changing the symptoms. Always try to keep things simple. One of the herbs in the formula is used to force the formula into the body, to keep it simple we will only use three, they are Licorice, Ginger and Cayenne.

As an example let's use an animal with a cough. After further study of the case we decide that this is a Acute Disease for it came on quick and is fast acting not slow like a Chronic Disease. Listening to the animals cough we decide that it is a dry cough and upon looking at the animals nose we can't see any mucus. Let's list the actions to consider.

Expectorants - Licorice, Aniseed, Fennel, Garlic and Mullein

Antispasmodics - Aniseed and Fennel

Demulcents - Licorice and Coltsfoot

Immune Boosters - Echinacea

Anti-Bacterial and Virals - Garlic and Echinacea

Out of the above I would choose Licorice, Echinacea, Garlic, Aniseed and Fennel. I would make the formula in this strength.

Formula
Licorice - 20%
Garlic - 15%
Echinacea - 15%
Aniseed - 30%
Fennel - 20%

Look these herbs up in the herbal and consider why I used them, there are three obvious ones for Licorice alone with the first being to force the assimilation of the formula into the body, second is its expectorant action and third is its demulcent action in case the throat is sore and raw. Next time you see a little kid eating heaps of licorice get them to open their mouth and look at their tongue which will be going black from the Licorice along with the throat etc and know that you are looking at the demulcent action of Licorice working by coating and soothing.

The most important reason that you use the Actions Method for Herbal Prescribing is so that you can concentrate the Actions which are most needed for example, if it's a Bacterial infection concentrate on the Anti Bacterials, if it's a Viral infection concentrate on the Anti Virals, hopefully you are now beginning to see the importance of working in actions for if you don't concentrate a large part of the battle on the causes you may have lost the battle from the start.

Read through all the Actions listed in Herbal Actions at the end of each body system in the book and then do a study in depth of at least five Actions of your choice making the first two the Anti Bacterials and Anti Virals. Start trying to train your mind into thinking in Actions.

How to Make Herbal Tinctures

Tinctures are made by steeping the Herb plant material in a mixture of alcohol and water. Alcohol is usually always used at astrength of 45%. The alcohol in this mixture will extract all the essential oils from the herb while the water will extract all that is water soluble, so between the both we are getting most of the medicinal properties out of the herb.

The proportions of herb to liquid are usually 1 part herb to 5 parts liquid. So find a suitable container (I use a big one liter preserving jar with a good sealing lid) and put into it 100grams of your chosen herb and to that add 500mls of our 45% solution of alcohol. Seal the lid and shake well for about a minute. Leave the jar on the window sill so the sun can shine on the jar for two weeks. The jar must be shaken for at least a minute every day.

After 2 weeks open and filter the contents of the jar. I use a large pouring jug into which I place a funnel and then place a coffee filter in the funnel and pour the jar contents through the funnel being careful not to let too much herb spill into the filter and block it up. When you get to the bottom of the jar you can crush the herb in your fist so as to extract the last of the liquid.

After this is completed you then get your chosen storage bottle, put a funnel into its neck followed by a coffee filter and then filter the jug into the bottle. Remember the solution should always be double filtered

Next we label the bottle, put the date, name and proportions eg 1 to 5 also state the recommended dose. Store in a cool and dark place. Most Professional Homoeopaths and Herbalists have access to pure alcohol so for them it is fairly easy to make tinctures while for the lay person they will probably have a hard time. A alternative is to use Vodka as strong as you can find it or find a way to twist the authorities arm into giving alcohol at 45%. Don't even try to get pure alcohol as it is dangerous and can turn people blind and they won't give it to you.

How to Make Infusions

Infusions are a bit like making a cup of tea except we don't use milk. Infusions are used for the soft parts of the herb such as the flowers, leaves and fine twigs. The proportions for infusions are 1 to 20 eg 1 part herb to 20 parts water. Infusions are used for the more water soluble herbs.

Infusions can be made from a single herb or from a combination of herbs and may be drunk hot or cold. The water should be just off the boil before being poured on the herb and if you are making a infusion of a herb strong in essential oils such as Peppermint always cover the top of the cup to stop the essential oils from escaping in steam while the infusion is brewing. Allow up to 10 minutes to brew. It is best to make herbal teas fresh each day. You can experiment on yourself by getting Chamomile and Peppermint tea bags from the supermarket. Use honey as a sweetener.

How to Make Decoctions

Decoctions are used for the more hard woody substances of the herb such as barks, berries or roots. The process of decoction is far more vigorous then infusion as it involves heating the plant material in cold water, bringing it to the boil and simmering for 20 to 40 minutes. The finished ratio for decoctions is again 1 part herb to 20 parts water, remember to add more water at the beginning so you wind up with the 1 to 20 after steam loss. This form of preparation is no good for the herbs that are high in essential oils as these will all be lost in the steam.

How to Make Poultices

Poultices are used to sooth, irritate or draw impurities from the skin so choose your required plants by the actions you need. A Poultice is used to apply a remedy to the skin with moist heat and slight pressure. To prepare a poultice bruise or crush the fresh medicinal parts of the herb you are using into a pulpy mass and add a little hot water if needed. If using dried herb moisten the material by mixing with a hot soft adhesive substance such as moist flower and cornmeal or as they did in the past a mixture of bread and milk. This can be done to the fresh herb if you want as well. For ease of application to the skin it is best to spread the mixture on cheese cloth and fold to the appropriate size or shape required. The cloth also helps by retaining the moisture and even allows you to tie it gently the affected area. Moisten the cloth with hot water periodically when and if needed. Hot water bottles can also be used to keep the poultice warm. Always keep some cloth between the skin when using irritant plants such as mustard and always wash the skin thoroughly after use.

Dosage For Forms Of Herbal

Medicines

Herbs can be given to animals in several different forms depending on what best suites the herb, the ailment, and the condition of the animal and of what is available at the time and then most importantly the expense.

Herbal Extract - Are alcohol based and about the strongest herbal preparation you can get as they nearly extract everything from the herb. Generally the strength is every ml should be equivalent to one gram of the herb. Used and dosed the same as tinctures but the dose will always be less than what is used in a tincture. From this try to work out if the extra price is worth it. Supplier should give dosage.

Tincture - Is a weaker then Herbal Extracts but also made from alcohol. Dilute the appropriate number of drops in water for treatment. Supplier should give dosage.

Infusion - A infusion is like making a cup of tea out of the flowers and leaves and other soft parts of the herb. Add boiling water and cover so as all the essential oils don't escape in the steam and leave for 20 minutes.

Decoction - Usually made from the root, bark or seed and is simmered for a while to extract the medicinal properties. Usually dosed the same as infusions.

Powdered - These are usually made from roots and bark and given in doses from a teaspoon to tablespoon. These can also be infused and turned into a tea. Try to get powdered extracts as they are more the real thing instead of for example powdered Ginger at the supermarket.

Fresh Herb - This is the easiest way to medicate a horse just add a large handful of the leaves to the feed. Always check for woody parts and sharp stalks. For dangerous or strong herbs chop finely and mix thoroughly into moistened feed so no one animal eats too much.

Dried Herb - Most dried herb is usually cut, again run your hand through for wood or sharps. If you are growing the herb yourself cut up or grind and mix directly with the feed. Crushed herbs can also be mixed with water and formed into a pill for individual treatment or the whole stable can be dosed in a mix with feed.

Note - Always be guided by the recommended dose of the individual herb instead of working in generals.

Calculating the Correct Dose for Animals

The Human dose is usually listed at the bottom of each herb to allow you to use the information below to find the right dose.

Cats - 1/8 to 1/6 the dose for an adult human.

Dogs - Correspond to adult human dose according to weight.

Horses - 8 to 16 times the dose for an adult human.

Goats - 2 times the dose for an adult human.

Sheep - 1 and a half times the dose for an adult human.

Cow - 12 to 24 times the dose for an adult human.

Swine - 1 to 3 times the dose for an adult human.

Not all herbs are of the same strength so for this reason it is a good idea to always look at the human dose and if this dose seems to be lower than normal, do your research into why. It might be a good idea to have a look at the herb Poke Root just to see what a strong herb looks like and can do.

Herbal General Animal Doses
Common Herbal Dosages for Herbivores from Dr Hue Karreman

Form	*Goat*	*Cow*	*Horse*
Decoction	4oz	12oz	8oz
Extract Powder	1 tsp	2tbs	2tbs
Extract Tablet	3 to 5	10 to 15	10 to 15
Tincture	1 tsp	2 tbs	2 - 3 tbs

Herbivores require less per pound relative to the human or carnivore

Dosage. These doses are given two to three times daily.

Tbsp. = Tablespoon, roughly = to 15cc

Dr. Hubert Karreman is a 1995 graduate from the University of Pennsylvania School of Veterinary Medicine. He has been a dairy practitioner for 16 years in Lancaster, Pennsylvania. He is an internationally recognized expert in the non-antibiotic treatment of infectious disease.

Sheep - For sheep I would give a slightly smaller dose then that of the Goat as sheep are less hardy and have been severely genetically changed as I was trying to point out with my cover on the Old Sheep book.

Warning - Not all herbs in nature are of the same strength. For example if you gave the very strong herb Poke Root in Calculating correct herbal doses for animals

Herbal

Agrimony

Actions - Astringent, cholagogue, diuretic, vulnerary, tonic

Used as a remedy for jaundice, it should be given to fasting animal as a drench or finely cut and mixed with bran; it is also a valuable astringent to stem bleeding and is a remedy for sore throats. Sprains are aided by a lotion made by boiling one handful of chopped Agrimony in one quart of brew made from wheaten bran. The combination of astringency and of bitter tonic properties make this a powerful herb for the digestive system. This is a good and gentle remedy for the young.

Uses - Diarrhea in the young, mucous colitis, spring tonic, indigestion, urinary incontinence and cystitis, as a gargle for sore throats and laryngitis and as a ointment or lotion for wounds and bruises.

For Cats and Dogs - Sore throats, Tonsillitis, infections of the mouth, Ailments of the lungs, stomach, liver kidney and bladder particularly cirrhosis of the liver and jaundice, it helps rheumatism, poor digestion and back pain and is excellent for enlargement of the heart and disorders of the spleen. Infusions, decoctions, ointments.

Human Dose - 1 to 3mls of tincture 3 times a day.

Cautions - Not to be used during Pregnancy

Alfalfa

Known also as Lucerne. Rich in nitrates and vitamins is a good tonic food and a kidney cleanser. Excellent for all animals and poultry. Fodder, tonic, nervine, aids in healing allergies, arthritis, morning sickness, peptic ulcers, stomach ailments and bad breath, removes poisons from the body, neutralizes acids, is a excellent blood purifier and thinner, improves appetite and aids in the assimilation of protein, calcium and other nutrients.

Cat - Half a teaspoon of alfalfa sprouts mixed into meals. Stops them from wanting to eat grass.

Dogs - 2 teaspoons of fresh chopped alfalfa sprouts with daily meal as a natural enzyme for good digestion.

Angelica

Actions - Expectorant, anti-spasmodic, diaphoretic, diuretic, carminative.

Useful expectorant for coughs, bronchitis and pleurisy especially when they are accompanied by fever, colds or influenza. The leaf can be used as a compress in inflammations of the chest. Its high oil content helps in intestinal colic and flatulence. Can ease rheumatic inflammations, in cystitis it acts as a urinary antiseptic.

Uses - Coughs, bronchitis, pleurisy, colic, wind, rheumatic inflammations, cystitis.

Human Dose - 2 to 5mls of tincture 3 times a day.

Aniseed

Actions - Expectorant, antispasmodic, carminative, parasiticide, aromatic.

Dogs like aniseed so much that it was once used as bait by dog thieves. As a carminative it is unsurpassed. An important remedy for all digestive ailments including colic.

Uses - Gripping, intestinal colic, wind, as a expectorant in bronchitis, tracheitis, irritable coughing, whooping cough

External - The oil by itself will help in the control of lice and scabies.

Human Dose – 1 cup of tea 3 times a day before meals.

Dose - Average dose is one handful of seeds daily. (Must be for larger animals)

Arnica

Actions - Anti-inflammatory, vulnerary.

For external use only Homoeopathic preparations can be used internally. For the treatment of shock and pains from accidents, bruises, joint stiffness and wounds, swellings, paralysis, sprains, rheumatic conditions or where ever there is inflammation on the skin. Use only as a lotion 1 to 20 externally on the skin. Do not use on broken skin or wounds.

Caution - Do not apply to open wounds or broken skin.

Homoeopathy - Used from 3C to 200C orally for injury, bleeding, bruising, shock or for any conditions that feel bruised or have a bruised like feeling.

Astragalus

Actions - Immuno-modulator, anti-viral, adaptogen, hypotensive, immune stimulant, adrenal tonic, diuretic, circulatory stimulant, vasodilator, blood tonic.

This herb should only be used in chronic diseases, as a preventative or in cases of fatigue especially in chronic diseases. Stimulates the natural production of interferon and intensifies the white cell destruction of germs.

A good tonic for strengthening the resistance to disease. Is very useful for animals in a state of chronic debility and fatigue by restoring the immune function. Use as a lung tonic to help expel toxins and pus in flu's, colds and sinusitis. Increases stamina and can accelerate wound healing, can help to replenish bone marrow. Strengthens the digestive system and aids adrenal gland function. This herb is used for cancer especially if the patient has had chemotherapy and helps aid them in their recovery.

This is a good herb to consider when animals have to travel, more so for livestock as it protects immunity, strengthens and preserves condition.

Uses - Boosting immune system, disease preventative, fatigue, healing wounds. This is a good herb to use before and during a long distance or time consuming transportation.

Human Dose - 500 to a 1000mg per day or up to 20drops of tincture twice daily.

Cautions - Should not be used in acute infections or fevers.

Barberry

Actions - Cholagogue, anti-emetic, bitter tonic, laxative, alterative, hypotensive, and antibacterial.

Good for correcting liver function and increasing the flow of bile. The herb is also a bitter tonic and mild laxative, use for weak and debilitated animals to strengthen and clean the system. Has been known to reduce enlarged spleens and also act against malaria. Its antibacterial properties have shown activity against strep, staph salmonella, shigella and eschorichia. This herb also dilates blood vessels thus lowering blood vessels.

Uses - Inflammation of the gallbladder, stones, liver problems, jaundice, arthritis, intestinal infections.

Cautions - Use only the dried plant and avoid during pregnancy.

Human Dose - Tincture 2 to 4mls three times daily

Bear Berry - Uva Ursi

Actions - Diuretic, astringent, antiseptic and demulcent.

Bear Berry has a specific antiseptic and astringent effect on the membranes of the urinary system and will generally soothe tone and strengthen them. It is specifically used where there is gravel or ulceration in the kidneys or bladder. A very useful herb where there is cystitis.

Uses - Urinary infections, gravel and ulcerations in the urinary system also to soothe these areas.

Human Dose - 2 to 4mls of tincture 3 times a day.

Black Cohosh

Actions - Emmenagogue, anti-spasmodic, alterative, sedative.

Has hormone balancing properties, encourages oestrogen production, good for pets that loose hair after being spayed, painful or delayed menstruation, ovarian cramps, cramping pain, used to regain normal hormone activity, rheumatoid and osteoarthritis, muscular and neuralgic pains.

Human Dose - 2 to 4mls of tincture 3 times daily.

Blue Flag

Actions - Cholagogue, alterative, laxative, diuretic, anti-inflammatory.

Often called liver lily which shows its use in liver ailments. It acts as a general conditioner for the whole system and is also a gentle laxative. Stimulates the digestive glands. This is usually used with other blood cleansers and should be used in small doses at first in case it stirs up too much rubbish.

Uses - Treatment of all liver ailments, jaundice, gall bladder disorders, general tonic, appetizer, mild laxative, eczema, skin diseases, psoriasis.

Human Dose - 2 to 4 mls of tincture 3 times a day.

Boswella

Actions - Anti-inflammatory, Ant arthritic, astringent

Good for use in any of the chronic inflammations in any body system.

Uses - Lung diseases especially of the chronic kind with inflammation, rheumatic diseases, diarrhea, dysentery, piles, STDs. It is also used in general weakness.

Human Dose - 200 to 400mg of extract three times daily.

Broom

Actions - Cardioactive diuretic, hypertensive, peripheral vasoconstrictor, astringent.

Russian peasants use Broom tops as a very successful remedy for rabies. It is also used as a mild vermifuge. The flowers infused in hot milk (one handful to one pint) are used internally and externally to cure severe forms of skin ailments. The young twigs are mildly purgative.

Uses - Worms, skin ailments, rabies, dropsy, constipation, increases flow of urine in kidney ailments, used where there is a weak heart and low blood pressure, profuse menstruation.

Human Dose - 1 to 2 mls of tincture 3 time a day.

Caution - Do not use in pregnancy and high blood pressure.

Burdock

Actions - Alterative, diuretic, bitter, antibacterial, anti-tumor.

It is used to treat conditions arising from an "overabundance" of toxins, such as boils, rashes and chronic skin problems. Helps to cleanse the body of waste products. Animals will not graze this herb with the exception of the ass, but the sliced and bruised roots are one of the finest blood cleansers known to herbalists. The bruised leaves applied externally are a remedy for ring worm and scabies. Soothing to the kidneys and an excellent diuretic. The juice is used internally for scabies and mites.

Uses - Remedy for all blood disorders, rheumatism, skin parasites , skin conditions resulting in dry scaly skin, psoriasis, eczema, dandruff, aids digestion and appetite, aids kidney function and helps with cystitis, speeds up the healing of wounds and ulcers. Use to reduce tumors.

Human Dose - 2 to 4 mls of tincture 3 times a day.

Horses - In powdered form begin with one teaspoon

full twice a day added to feed and can be increased to 2 teaspoons full twice a day if needed.

Buchu

Actions - Diuretic, urinary antiseptic, digestive tonic, kidney tonic.

Used in any infection of the genito-urinary system such as cystitis, urethritis and prostatitis. Especially useful in painful and burning urination. Good kidney tonic. Used to treat blood in the urine, stones and chronic urinary infections especially if started by colon bacteria.

Human Dose - 2 to 4mls of tincture 3 times a day.

Cayenne

Actions - Stimulant, carminative, tonic, sialagogue, rubefacient, anti-septic.

Used as a catalyst to help push herbal formulas into the body. Aids heart failure (a few drops on the side of the mouth), stimulates the heart, helps heal ulcers of the stomach and colon, cayenne powder sprinkled on a open wound stops bleeding, flatulent dyspepsia, colic. Externally it is used as a rubefacient in problems like lumbago and rheumatic pains.

Human Dose - 0.25 to 1ml of tincture 3 times daily or when needed.

Caution - High doses on an empty stomach can cause gut irritation and eventually ulcers

Calendula

Actions - Anti-inflammatory, astringent, vulnerary, anti-fungal, cholagogue, emmenagogue.

Goats and sheep seek it out; the flowers are tonic and a good heart medicine they possess restorative powers over the arteries and veins, the flowers are also fed to make miserable fretting animals cheerful, also used for liver problems, vomiting, internal ulcers.

Uses - Cuts, grazes, infected sores, fungal infections, any skin inflammations, regulates the oil production of the skin so is good for acne, to stop bleeding, bruises and sprains, skin ulcers and minor burns and scolds, healing, soothing, anti-microbial. Use as a lotion to clean wounds, one of our main germacides for wounds and if Hypericum is added to the lotion you may prevent tetanus as well.

Human Dose - Use internally as a cholagogue, for Candida, gallbladder problems, ulcers, indigestion, painful periods, delayed menstruation - Dose 1 to 4 mls of tincture 3 times daily. Use externally as a lotion (1 to 20) or a cream.

Caution - Calendula closes wounds rapidly so make sure they are very clean and no foreign bodies remain.

Cat Mint (Cat Nip)

Actions - Carminative, antispasmodic, diaphoretic, sedative, astringent.

This herb is also known as Catnip. Cats and other creatures eat this plant and also give themselves a massage in it. This plant sometimes causes cats to grow pensive and dreamy. This is an old traditional cold and flu remedy especially ones with fever. Has an action on the digestive system easing stomach upsets, dyspepsia, wind and colic. Used for diarrhea of the young. Good for nervous, stressed or restless animals.

Human Dose - 2 to 4mls of tincture 3 times a day.

Cats Claw

Actions - Anti oxidant, immune stimulant, anti-inflammatory, anti-fungal, anti-rheumatic, anti-viral, anti-tumor, anti-microbial.

To alleviate allergic sinus type conditions, boost the immune system, asthma, bursitis, Candida, immune deficiency disorders, chronic inflammatory diseases, auto immune conditions.

Human Dose - 30 to 75ml per week

Cautions - Dont use during pregnancy.

Celery Seed

Actions - Anti rheumatic, diuretic, carminative, sedative, alterative, hypotensive.

The main use for this herb is in the treatment of rheumatism, arthritis and gout. Celery seed can help soothe the nerves and relieve pain and also aids the body in the removal of uric acid. A good cleansing, mildly diuretic herb, useful in ridding the system of an accumulation of waste products. An improvement in circulation of fluids encourages a horse to drink and sweat more easily. Celery seed mixed with food aids in the digestion of protein. A very good digestive tonic if the horse is run down with little appetite.

Uses - Arthritis, hyperacidity, pain, hypertension, digestion, urinary tract infections

Human Dose - 2 to 4mls of tincture 3 times daily.

Horses- 1 tablespoon twice daily.

Caution - Not to be used with kidney diseases or during pregnancy.

Centaury

Actions - Bitter, aromatic, mild nervine, gastric stimulant, chologogue, febrifuge, vermafuge.

Use whenever a gastric stimulant is required especially in cases of anorexia and liver weakness. This is a good herb for use in the young.

Uses - For digestive ailments, jaundice, as a vermafuge including liver fluke, use externally for lice, wounds and warts. In the past it was also used as a birth remedy.

Human Dose - 1 to 2 mls of tincture 3 times daily, best 20 minutes before meals.

Chamomile

Actions - Carminative, sedative, anti-spasmodic, anti-inflammatory, analgesic and anti-septic.

It is a famed blood cleanser and pain reducer, reduces tumors (poultice), remedy for female ailments, inflamed gums, use for blood and skin disorders, aches and pains, external and internal inflammations, delayed menstruation, acid uterus and all female ailments, cleanser and toner of the digestive tract, it is well documented as having anti-inflammatory activity and is also beneficial in reducing allergic responses as it contains a number of anti-histamine chemicals. In addition, it is recognized as being ulcer-protective through its healing effect on the mucosa of the gastro-intestinal tract, expels worms and parasites, improves and helps appetite. Good for nervous and hyperactive horses as it calms them without making them tired.

Uses - Indigestion, colic, diarrhea, teething, anxiety, insomnia, nervous upsets, slowing down hyperactive horses, flatulence. Good all round tonic for the nervous system especially for nervous animals.

Cats and Dogs - Good for kittens and puppies, administer in all cases of stomach pain, wind, upsets, gastritis, restlessness and fever. Can be given also for all abdominal and uterine disorders, inflammation of the testicles, wounds, toothaches, eruptions and as a steam bath for colds and feline respiratory diseases. Fevers, back and rheumatic pains are eased by the tea and regular massages with the oil. The infusion is good for nervous disorders and a tonic for kidney and urinary tract problems

Horses -1 cup of infusion added to feed twice a day or a hand full of flowers replacing the infusion.

Human Dose - 2 to 4mls 3 times daily.

Chaparral

Actions - Alterative, astringent, diuretic, tonic, powerful antioxidant, anti-arthritic, anti-rheumatic, anti-cancer, anti-tumor, dissolves calculi, anti-biotic.

Uses - Used in kidney problems and stones and for rheumatism and arthritis. Aids in healing skin blemishes, acne, allergies, promotes hair growth, acts as a natural anti-biotic, cataracts, has a action on cancer.

Human Dose - 10 to 30 drops a day.

Chaste Tree

Actions - Emmenagogue, galactagogue, Tonic for the reproductive organs.

More of a hormone balancer by working directly on the pituitary gland though is more of a normalizing herb, usually increases the progesterone levels therefore increasing the chance of pregnancy. Supporting the progesterone level is extremely helpful in counteracting the irritability and unpredictability that can happen with mares in season making them more comfortable, cooperative and safer to handle. Though this herb is primarily used to balance hormonal irregularities in mares it can also be used to inhibit the sex hormones of stallions if their behavior is thought dangerous or seen to be causing them a loss in condition. Useful on its own or in combination with herbs specific for hormonal balance.

Used for endometriosis, fibroids, infertility and threatened miscarriages.

Human Dose – 1 to 2mls of tincture 3 times daily

Chickweed

Actions - Healing, anti-inflammatory, astringent, emollient.

Rich in copper, highly tonic food for the digestive system and a remedy for all stomach ailments, allergies, colon problems, constipation, piles, rheumatism, skin problems, eczema, psoriasis, itching, irritation, cuts and wounds.

Uses - One of the main uses of this herb is for itching skin conditions whether from insect bites or eczema like conditions. Has wound healing and demulcent properties.

Dose - Usually given in infusions or used as a lotion or cream.

Cleavers

Actions - Alterative, diuretic, anti-inflammatory, astringent, tonic, anti-cancer.

A lymphatic tonic with alterative and diuretic actions which can be used in a wide range of problems where the lymphatic system is involved. The plant is very rich in minerals and silica, gives good strong texture to the hair of animals, eggs and strengthens the hoofs. Also used to ease swollen legs and joints, support the lymphatic and endocrine systems and encourage the elimination of toxins, is also helpful if your horse experiences muscle tightening during or after exercise. All animals eat it and poultry especially seek it hence its popular name of goose grass. Good for skin ailments.

Cats and Dogs - Cleavers is a great purifier of the kidneys, pancreas and spleen. Disorders of the uterus, the lymphatic system and the skin are helped by this herb. The fresh juice applied to cases of feline acne and eczema quickly alleviates the problem as do regular washings of the infected areas with cleavers tea. Washes can also be used on wounds and abscesses. Internal treatment can be used for epilepsy, anemia, dropsy, nervous complaints and constriction of the vocal cords. Toms suffering from a blocked bladder will be greatly helped by a regular dose of cleavers as the tea dissolves gravely deposits in the bladder. Cancer of the tongue and mouth and other cancerous growths are helped.

Uses - Tonic, eczema, abscesses and tumors, cancerous growths, swollen glands, tonsillitis, psoriasis, cystitis.

Horses - 1 cup full daily or 2 tablespoons full of powder daily.

Human Dose - 2 to 4mls of tincture 3 times a day.

Coltsfoot

Actions - Expectorant, anti tussive, demulcent, anti-catarrhal, diuretic.

The Latin name means banish cough.. Coltsfoot combines a soothing expectorant action with a anti-spasmodic action. There are useful zinc levels in this plant. Consider this herb in any respiratory problem.

Cats and Dogs - Most particularly a chest herb with powerful expectorant and anti-inflammatory properties. Excellent for cases of bronchitis, bronchial asthma, pleurisy, Feline Respiratory Disease and chest problems that accompany a range of feline fungal diseases. It can be given with honey and lemon when coughing is a persistent problem. Can be used as a poultice for non-healing wounds. Ear infections can be helped by the fresh juice.

Uses - Coughs, pneumonia, asthma, pleurisy, TB, sedative powers in epilepsy, chronic or acute bronchitis, emphysema, cystitis.

Externally - A poultice is used for abscess, ulcers, boils, earache and toothache.

Human Dose - (illegal in Australia) 2 to 4mls of

tincture 3 times daily.

Comfrey

Actions - Demulcent, astringent, healing, expectorant.
Once widely cultivated as a fodder plant, sheep and cows eat it greedily, the impressive wound healing powers of comfrey are partially due to allantoin which stimulates cell proliferation and speeds the healing process inside and out. Has been used for thousands of years as a herb with abilities to mend broken bones. Has the same result on wounds, tendons, fractures, sprains, ulcers and cartilage.

Cats and Dogs - One of the best wound and bone setting herbs. The tincture is effective of curing rheumatism and swollen joints even where arthritis has caused extensive damage. The tincture has been used for paralysis. Massage well into the joints and muscles of the affected parts. Where paralysis is due to shock, dislocation or sprain, apply as a poultice. A cold infused tisane prepared overnight from the roots is good for digestive ailments, bronchitis, internal bleeding in the stomach, lungs or bowels, pleurisy and internal ulcers.

Uses - Its old name is knit bone and that describes well what it does. Comfrey also guards against scar tissue from developing incorrectly, all internal hemorrhages including uterine, reunion of wound and fractures, internal ulcers, ruptures, pulmonary problems, bronchitis, irritable cough, ulcerative colitis, skin ulcers and varicose veins.

Horses - Half a cup of the cut herb up to 3 times daily.

Human Dose - 2 to 4mls 3 times daily.

Corn Silk

Actions - Diuretic, demulcent, tonic, antiseptic, antilithic.

A soothing diuretic that is helpful in any irritation of the membranes of the urinary system. Combined with other herbs in the treatment of cystitis, urethritis and prostatitis. Cleanses and soothes the urinary system.

Cats and Dogs - Good for the treatment of obesity and as it is a powerful diuretic it can be used for all complaints of the bladder and kidneys especially stones, edema, fluid in the heart, nephritis, cystitis, renal colic, and rheumatism.

Human Dose - 3 to 6mls of tincture 3 times a day.

Cranesbill

Action - Strong astringent, anti-inflammatory, vulnerary.

One of the best astringents known for internal and external use and is palatable to most animals.

Uses - Dysentery and diarrhea especially in the old and young, piles, duodenal or gastric ulcers, uterine hemorrhage or any internal bleeding especially of the digestive and respiratory systems, douche in leucorrhoea, treatment of wounds.

Human Dose - 2 to 4 mls of tincture 3 times daily

Cranberry

Actions - Urinary antiseptic

Cranberry inhibits the adhesion of bacteria to the urinary pipe lines so each time water is passed the bacteria is flushed out thus preventing recolonization.

Human Dose - Use doses from 5000 to 15000mg. Use strong doses for acute infection and smaller doses as a preventative.

Dandelion

Actions - Diuretic, cholagogue, anti-rheumatic, laxative, tonic

The leaves of the Dandelion plant are generally fed to horses during spring as the herb assists with cleansing the blood. They are high in iron and calcium as well as Vitamins A, B, and D and are traditionally used as a tonic to stimulate the bladder.

The herb is blood cleansing and tonic, it has an important effect on the hepatic system and is a supreme jaundice curative herb, the leaves strengthen the enamel of the teeth and the white juices of the freshly crushed stem dissolves warts, the plant is well grazed by goats, horses will take quantities of the leaves when cut and well mixed with bran. Dandelion Root is helpful for horses recovering from an illness or a reaction to vaccination. Being a tonic, this herb assists to clean the liver, kidneys and blood and is high in potassium and magnesium. Excellent for anemia because it is high in iron, calcium, copper and vitamins, useful in kidney and bladder problems, skin eruptions, sluggish blood flow, weak arteries, all liver complaints, jaundice, constipation, gallbladder problems and rheumatism.

Horses - 2 tablespoons of powder daily or make as infusion and pour over feed.

Cats and Dogs - A good liver herb especially for gall bladder complaints. It can be used for eczema and feline miliary dermatitis and is a healing tonic for the spleen. Internal digestive toning and cleansing along with metabolic disorders.

Human Dose - 5 to 10 mls of tincture 3 times daily.

Devils Claw

Actions - Anti-inflammatory, pain killer, hepatic, anti-rheumatic, alterative.

Used for its analgesic and anti-inflammatory properties, it is useful for treating pain in a range of joint and muscular problems. The bitter action of Devils Claw stimulates and tones the digestive system. Good for reducing inflammation in arthritis, gout and rheumatism. Aids the body in the elimination of uric acid. This plant also aids liver and gallbladder complaints.

Horses - 1 tablespoon of powder twice a day or more in severe conditions but only for a short time.

Human Dose - 1 to 2mls of tincture 3 times daily.

Caution - Use with demulcent herbs to save irritating the tummy, don't use on horses with ulcers.

Dong Quai

Actions - Emmenagogue, antispasmodic, analgesic, uterine tonic ,vasodilator, hormone balancer, alterative.

Known regulator for the female reproductive system. Some of its compounds stimulate the uterus while others relax the uterus. The compounds that stimulate the uterus are water soluble and are absorbed into the body from teas and capsules. The compounds that relax the uterus are soluble in alcohol and are provided by tinctures. This herb may stop cramping, and ease the pain of ovarian cysts. The Chinese use this herb for abnormal menstruation, suppressed flow, painful or difficult menstruation. This herb is also good for the treatment of psoriasis. Dong Quai also helps with , asthma, bronchitis, emphysema and improves the function of the lungs. Builds and improves circulation as well as disperses congestion in the pelvic area.

Human Dose - 6 to 18 grams of dried root per day and in the tablet form 1500mg per day.

Horses - 1 to 3 teaspoon full per day depending on severity of the condition.

Cautions - Avoid during pregnancy and in cases with diarrhea and dysentery.

Echinacea

Actions - Immune stimulant, anti-microbial, anti-inflammatory, alterative, healing.

Is an infection fighter active against strep bacteria (abscesses and boils), a blood cleanser, (blood poisons, snake bites, poisonous insects) and a glandular and lymphatic system cleanser. Use it particularly for respiration infections and for any disease above the waist. This is one of our main immune boosters for the acute diseases. Use as a prophylactic to protect horses and livestock from infections especially when traveling. When traveling add Astragalus.

Uses - All infections, depressed immune function, inflammatory conditions, allergies, effective against both bacteria and viruses.

Human Dose - 1 to 4mls of tincture three times daily. For cats 3 drops twice daily in food.

Horses - half to 1 tablespoon 3 times daily or half a cup dry leaf or shaved root up to 3 times daily depending on the severity of the condition. Infusions can be used to.

Warning - Do not use continually as you will burn out the immune system, for chickens because of their faster metabolism use no longer than 3 weeks but start with a reasonably strong dose. Beware also in the use of allergies for you could be building up the immune system just to attack itself.

Elecampane

Actions - Expectorant, antitussive, anti-bacterial, antifungal, diaphoretic, stomachic, demulcent.

This herb is meant to be named after Helen of Troy and is a very ancient herb used for thousands of years especially by the Romans. Specific for irritating bronchial coughs, lots of catarrh, has a soothing and anti-bacterial action.

Mainly used for treating chronic coughs, bronchitis and asthma especially in the young. . It is also used for digestive problems. Elecampane also contains Alantolactone which helps to expel intestinal parasites such as pin worm. A external wash can help deter Scabies.

Uses - Bronchitis, emphysema, asthma and digestive problems. In the past was used for TB.

Human Dose - 1 to 2mls of tincture 3 times a day.

Elder

Actions - Diaphoretic, diuretic, anti-catarrhal, expectorant.

Most animals will graze on elder. Used for the treatment of all gastric, hepatic, and pulmonary ailments, all fevers, skin disorders especially scabies and ring worm, externally as an insecticide.

Leaves - Externally emollient and vulnerary (bruises, sprains and wounds). Internally used as a purgative, expectorant, diuretic and Diaphoretic. Topically the lotion makes a anti-inflammatory wash, salve, eyewash and gargle for sore throats.

Flowers - Diaphoretic and Anti catarrhal. Use for colds and flu.

Berries - Diaphoretic and Anti catarrhal. The uses are similar to the flowers but the berries are used for rheumatism. The berries have been used as a nutrient rich tonic given after birth to help build the blood.

Dose - Really depends on which part of the plant you are using the leaves, flowers or berries. The tincture made of flowers is 2 to 4mls 3 times daily.

Eye Bright

Actions - Anti-inflammatory, astringent, anti-catarrhal.

As the name says this is one of the main herbs in the treatment of eye problems. The aerial (above ground) parts of the plant are used. As its name suggests, it helps eye problems by relieving inflammation and tightening mucous membranes and is specifically used in treating conjunctivitis and blepharitis. Used for infections and allergic conditions affecting the eyes, middle ear, sinuses and nasal passages.

The plant is also nervine, tonic and astringent. Its use is both internal and external strengthening greatly the eyes nerves when used so. The high potassium and sulphur content of the plant make it also of value in treatment of gastric ailments especially insufficiency of gastric juices. Acts as an internal medicine for the constitutional tendency to eye weakness.

Uses- Best known for its use in the eye where it is helpful in acute or chronic inflammations, stinging and weeping eyes, over sensitivity to light, conjunctivitis, allergies, sinusitis, ulcers and general eye weakness.

Human Dose - 1 to 4mls 3 times daily of tincture.

Horses - 1 teaspoon of powdered herb or half a cup of dried herb morning and night.

Fennel

Actions - Carminative, aromatic, anti-spasmodic, stimulant, galactagogue, expectorant.

The herb possesses highly antiseptic and tonic properties. The primary use of fennel is to relieve bloating, but it also settles stomach pain, stimulates the appetite and is diuretic and anti-inflammatory. Peasants drive their flocks to feed upon it owing to the abundance of milk that the herb produces and the sweet odor that it imparts upon the milk. (if the animal is not native they can over gorge and poison themselves).

Arabs use fennel poultices to resolve old and hard tumors.

Uses - Gastric ailments, relieves flatulence and colic, stimulates appetite, inflammation of the bowels, acute constipation (raw roots daily), fevers, cramps, worms, indigestion, all eye ailments, bronchitis, coughs, muscular and rheumatic pains use the oil. Externally used as an eye wash to treat eye infections.

Human Dose - 2 to 4mls of tincture 3 times daily.

Horses - One tablespoon of seeds given twice daily.

Fenugreek

Actions - Expectorant, demulcent, tonic, carminative, galactagogue, alterative, restorative.

Strongly aromatic herb and the seeds of the plant are used. It contains a volatile oil, flavonoids, mucilage, protein, Vitamins A, B & C, alkaloids, saponins and some minerals. The seeds can aid in recovery from illness and to encourage weight gain. This is a herb well worth getting to know not just because of its tonic properties but for its rubbish removing actions especially in mucous thick chronic diseases such as sinusitis. Always use cleansing herbs like this one slowly and at low doses especially when using for long periods of time. The plant possesses highly aromatic seeds having a powerful disinfectant, emollient and lubricant properties. The feeding value of these is about equal to linseed. It is one of the great fattening herbs. The perfect sister herb for garlic enhancing all its powers. Very tonic and eagerly sought by all animals. Rich in vitamins and nitrates, calcium and phosphorus. The whole plant is used.

Uses - Treatment for all gastric weaknesses and ailments, nerves and neuralgia, female ailments including failing milk supply, allergies, bronchitis, anemia, bruises, colitis, coughs, diabetes, fever, flu, hay fever, headache, migraines, lung problems, sinus congestion, ulcers, reduces inflammation, has a reputation for stimulating and developing breasts.

Externally - It can be used as a poultice for relief of abscess, boils, tumors and running sores.

Human Dose - Tincture 1 to 2mls of tincture three times a day. Or one to two handfuls of plant feed a day, to obtain a quicker result use the seed - 2 ounces of seed daily. Use seed for the poultices.

Horses - One to two handfuls of plant feed a day, to obtain a quicker result use the seed - 2 tablespoons of seed daily. Use seed for the poultices.

Caution - Avoid during pregnancy as it can be a uterine stimulant.

Feverfew

Actions - Anti-inflammatory, vasodilator, relaxant, digestive bitter, uterine stimulant.

It is one of the most important aids for female ailments the plant exerting remarkable powers over the uterus, the whole plant is used. Has a good reputation for migraine headaches, may help with arthritis when it is in the inflammatory stage, painful periods. Feverfew inhibits the manufacture of substances causing inflammation.

Uses - Digestive aid and tonic, treatment for all female irregularities especially scanty or failing menses, inflamed or weak uterus and uterine and vaginal ulcers, abortion, difficult labor, retained afterbirth, arthritis, inflammations.

Human Dose - 3 to 4mls 3 times daily.

Cautions - Do not use during pregnancy because of the stimulant action on the womb. The fresh leaves may cause mouth ulcers in sensitive people.

Figwort

Actions - Alterative, diuretic, mild purgative, heart stimulant.

Used for any skin condition where there is itching and irritation. This herb cleans out the system especially the blood and bowels. Can be used has a heart stimulant or for poor circulation but is contraindicated for this when there is a rapid heartbeat (tachycardia)

Uses - Failing or weak heart, eczema, psoriasis, acne, cradle cap, mild laxative. Externally use for boils, burns ,eczema, rashes, ringworm and wounds.

Human Dose - 2 to 4mls of tincture three times daily.

Fumitory

Actions - Diuretic, cholagogue, laxative, alterative.

Has a long history of use in the treatment of skin problems such as eczema and acne, its action is probably due to a general cleansing mediated via the kidneys and liver. Cows and sheep seek it out greedily. The whole plant is used.

Uses - All forms of liver ailments and gallbladder

problems, skin eruptions, eczema, wounds, scabies, ulcerated mouth, inflamed liver, jaundice, biliousness.

Human Dose - 1 to 2mls of tincture 3 times daily.

Garlic

Actions - Immune stimulant, anti-bacterial, anti-viral, anti-fungal, anti-septic, anti-oxidant, diaphoretic, cholagogue, hypotensive, anti-spasmodic, vermifuge and many more.

The plant is rich in volatile oil and sulphur and because of its remarkable penetrating, disinfecting and mucous expelling powers garlic is a valuable basic remedy for the treatment of all ailments in which the cleansing of the blood stream and expulsion of mucous accumulations is required. Garlic can be used to prevent and treat respiratory infections. Anyone who has had garlic breath has experienced this herb's aromatic compounds being excreted through their lungs which is why garlic's active ingredients can be so effective for respiratory complaints. Garlic is extremely effective in dissolving and cleansing cholesterol from the blood stream, it stimulates the digestive tract, kills worms, parasites and harmful bacteria, normalizes blood pressure, reduces fever, gas and cramps.

Uses- All infections, coughs, colds, flu, bronchitis, all fevers, pulmonary conditions, gastric and skin complaints, rheumatism, all worms and also liver fluke, mange, ringworm, ticks and lice.

Acts on Bacteria, Viruses and Internal Parasites.

Human Dose - 1 clove 3 times a day.

Horses - 1 clove every second day as maintenance. Two cloves a day in sickness but for only a couple of weeks.

Dogs - Crushed fresh garlic half a clove for small dog 1 clove for medium to large dog, crush and add to meals. Use in short bursts for dogs not exceeding a month in any 3 month period as it is now thought garlic can cause dog anemia so use for the acute diseases.

Externally - You can use garlic for ring worm and ear ache, to disinfect wounds and sores, parasitical infections.

Guaiacum

Actions - Anti rheumatic, anti-inflammatory, laxative, diaphoretic, diuretic, alterative, peripheral circulatory stimulant.

Specific for rheumatic complaints with lots of inflammation, aids in the treatment of gout and can be used here as a preventative. Care must be taken with this herb especially in allergic conditions.

Human Dose - 1 to 4mls of tincture 3 times a day.

Gentian

Actions - Bitter, gastric stimulant, sialagogue, cholagogue.

The root is the medicinal part. Gentian is one of the most important tonic herbs being considered the Prince of the Bitters. Quells vomiting when all other herbs fail, promotes the production of saliva, gastric juices and bile along with stimulating peristalsis, indicated where there is a lack of appetite and sluggishness of the digestive system.

Uses - Treatment of all forms of digestive weakness, vomiting, nervous ailments including hysteria, malaria, to improve the appetite of all poor feeders.

Human Dose - 1 to 4 mls of tincture 3 times a day. Dose 20 minutes before meals if using as a digestive.

Ginger

Actions - Carminative, anti-inflammatory, vasodilator, circulatory stimulant, diaphoretic, anti-emetic.

The therapeutic benefits of ginger are largely due to its volatile oil and oleoresin content. Ginger is an excellent remedy for many digestive complaints, including nausea, colic, wind and indigestion. Its antiseptic properties also make it beneficial for gastro-intestinal infections. For the older, arthritic horse, ginger is a useful maintenance herb. It stimulates the circulatory system and helps blood flow and increases stamina. Aids in fighting colds, colitis, digestive disorders, wind, increases saliva.

Uses- Indigestion, nausea, feverish conditions especially when chills are present, travel sickness especially sea sickness, dyspepsia, colic, flatulence.

Human Dose - Weak tincture 1.5 to 3mls 3 times daily.

Horse - In powder form 1 tablespoon twice a day or 1 tablespoon of grated 3 times a day or an infusion over feed 3 times a day.

Caution - Don't use large doses on an empty stomach.

Ginkgo Biloba

Actions - Anti fungal, anti-bacterial, antioxidant, anti tussive, astringent, expectorant, anti-allergy and anti-inflammatory but mainly used for its Peripheral Vaso - Dilator effects.

Is native to Northern China and is considered the world's oldest tree species. This herb can be helpful for a horse resuming work after a spell, or for older horses that are sound for riding but are slowing down. Due to its effect on peripheral and cerebral (brain) circulation it can assist the blood supply to limbs, and general alertness. (Think of mixing with Hawthorn). The leading symptoms pointing to Ginkgo are cold hands and feet. This herb opens up the femoral arteries and neck arteries increasing blood supply to those areas thus improving the function of everything in those areas by the increase in oxygen and blood sugar. For the old animal thinking and seeing may improve and walking may also become a bit easier. In asthma ginkgo helps reduce the inflammation response making the attacks less severe. The herb is safe to use as a tonic. This is a good herb to take in a mixed antioxidant formula.

Human Dose - 140 to 240mg extract per day.

Horse - 1 cup full twice daily of the cut leaf.

Ginseng (Panax)

Actions - Anti depressive, restorative, tonic, adaptogen, stimulating adrenal agent, increases resistance and improves mental and physical performance.

This is the strong ginseng, think twice about giving it to a horse with a shy and sensitive nature it's more for the outgoing and competitive nature. This herb can help with depression especially when caused by debility and exhaustion. It can be used in general for exhaustion and weakness. Used to increase mental and physical performance, to improve concentration, vigilance and work efficiency, stamina, for combating internal or external stress factors of any kind - athletics, endurance activities, aging, surgery, disease, infections, cold, but especially degenerative conditions and problems of old age. This is a good herb for infertility.

Human Doses - For the elderly and long term 400 to 800mgs per day. Short term 600 to 2000mg per day for 3 to 4 weeks then have a break for 4 weeks then you can go back on it if you wish. Remember month on month off as this herb can build up in the system.

During your month off you will still be getting the benefits of this herb as the excess leaves the body.

Horse - 1 teaspoon full of powdered herb and see what happens.

Cautions - Avoid with high blood pressure, during acute infections. This herb can be over stimulating for some. Use month on month off.

Ginseng Siberian

Actions - Adaptogen, vaso dilator, increases stamina, circulatory stimulant.

This herb is very similar to the one above but is a milder version and can be used all the time as it does not build up in the system like Panax Ginseng. Always consider giving a break from herbs as it is not good to use any herb all the time except maybe Hawthorn for a failing heart.

Human Dose – Maybe 500mg twice daily.

Horse - 1 teaspoon full in the feed up to 3 times a day.

Goldenrod

Actions - Anticatarrhal, anti-inflammatory, antiseptic, diaphoretic, carminative, diuretic, astringent, tonic, hypotensive.

It is famed as a wound herb, is a important remedy for female disorders, all cattle eat it and it brings them into good appetite and gives bloom, the whole plant is used, traditionally used for inflammation, upper respiratory catarrh, use with other herbs for influenza, flatulent dyspepsia, as a urinary anti-inflammatory and anti-septic, cystitis, urethritis and also used for urinary stones. This herb is also used for arthritis.

Cat and Dog - The blossoms are gathered to treat intestinal ulceration and bleeding of the intestines as well as dysentery, vomiting and flatulence. Leaves and flowers are used for kidney complaints as well as urinary and bladder problems.

Uses - A powerful digestive aid, treatment of jaundice, kidney problems.

Externally - For wounds, to stop bleeding, cleansing gangrenous conditions.

Human Dose - 2 to 4mls of tincture 3 times a day.

Gravel Root

Actions - Diuretic, anti-lithic, anti-rheumatic.

Used primarily for kidney stones and gravel. In urinary infections such as cystitis and urethritis it may be used with benefit, good in the systemic treatment of rheumatism and gout.

Human Dose - 1 to 2mls of tincture 3 times a day.

Grindelia

Actions - Antispasmodic, expectorant, hypotensive, cardiac relaxant, diuretic, tonic.

This plant comes from the Americas and has long been used for asthma; it acts to relax the smooth muscles and is good for asthma and bronchitis especially when these are associated with a rapid heartbeat and a nervous disposition. Also used for whooping cough and respiratory catarrh. Ellingwood a famous Herbalist from the past considered it a specific for asthmatic breathing. Because of the relaxing effect on the heart and pulse there may be a lowering of blood pressure. Has a tonic effect on the lungs and kidneys and is mildly diuretic.

Topically this herb has been used for eczema, insect bites, poison ivy and burns.

Human Dose - 1 to 2mls of tincture 3 times a day.

Caution - Don't use for those with weak hearts or low blood pressure.

Hawthorn

Actions - Cardiac tonic, hypotensive, adaptogen.

Strengthens the muscles and nerves of the heart, aids in relieving emotional stress, regulates high and low blood pressure, helps combat arteriosclerosis and heart disease. With regard to horses, hawthorn's affects on peripheral circulation makes it valuable for treating conditions such as navicular and laminitis. Indeed, horses and ponies suffering from these ailments have been observed seeking out the new growth on hawthorn bushes. This is more of a balancing herb, if the blood pressure is high or low the herb will balance it if the electrical activity is playing up with rapid or erratic heart beat it will try to balance it. Strengthens and helps to remove plaques from the blood vessels. This is an herb for taking in the long term.

Uses - As a tonic to the circulatory system and to strengthen the heart.

Human Dose - 2 to 4mls of tincture 3 times a day.

Horse - 2 tablespoons of the powdered berry 3 times daily mix in the feed.

Hops

Actions - Sedative, hypnotic, antiseptic, astringent, nervine, bitter digestive tonic, antibacterial.

Famed for its tonic and nervine properties, pain reliever, sleep inducer, anti-septic, vermifuge, tension that leads to restlessness, headache, indigestion, mucous colitis. Good for when digestive problems are caused by worry or nerves. Good for nervous horses. One of the main remedies for IBS. Acts on the central nervous system and calms and eases anxiety. Hops contains estrogenic substances which could interfere with hormone therapy.

Uses - Treatment of all digestive ailments, general debility, failing appetite, wasting, fevers, eczema, worms, to quietens restless animals.

Externally - Eczema.

Human Dose - 1 to 4mls of tincture 3 times daily.

Horehound (White)

Actions - Expectorant, anti-spasmodic, bitter, digestive, vulnerary.

Is one of the most important pectoral herbs a famed cough and throat remedy, the bitter action stimulates the flow of bile and thus improves digestion.

Uses - Treatment of cough, pneumonia, pleurisy, bronchitis, TB, atrophy of the lungs, ear disorders, canker, diarrhea, inflammation of the liver, jaundice.

Human Dose - 1 to 2mls of tincture 3 times a day.

Horse Chestnut

Actions - Circulatory tonic, astringent, anti-inflammatory, nutritive.

Has an action on the vessels of the circulatory system especially veins where it seems to increase their strength and tone. Can be used internally and externally on the veins themselves. The nuts in the past were fed to animals as a tonic food and was also said to enrich the milk. It also was used in the past to treat the cough of horses and this is where it gets its name.

Uses - Inflammation of veins, varicose veins, piles, capillary weakness

Human Dose - 1 to 4mls of tincture 3 times daily.

Cautions - Avoid with kidney disease.

Horseradish

Actions - Stimulant, carminative, mild laxative, diuretic, antiseptic, tonic.

It's hot properties make it valuable in expelling worms, stimulating appetite and as a general tonic, it is an internal antiseptic, helps to remove excess urine from the system and stones from the bladder, urinary infection, all parts of the plant are used, can be used in influenza and fevers, eases wind and gripping pains in the digestive system, bronchitis.

Uses - Worm and kidney treatment, to reduce tumors, asthma, bronchitis, sinusitis, remedy for lack of appetite and over thinness.

Externally - As a poultice for swellings.

Human Dose - Infusion of 1 teaspoon to 1 cup.

Horsetail

Actions - Astringent, diuretic, vulnerary.

Goats eat the plant but it is not a good food for cows, excellent astringent for the genito-urinary system reducing bleeding and healing wounds thanks to its high silica content, inflammation of the prostrate, tones and astringes the urinary system making it a good remedy for incontinence and bed wetting. Use for kidney stones as the high silica content erodes stones. May speed up the healing of bone, flesh and cartilage due to its high mineral content.

Cats and Dogs - Good for stopping internal

bleeding and vomiting of blood. Used for kidney and bladder problems, gravel and stones.

Uses - Nasal hemorrhage, laryngitis, intestinal ulcer, inflammation of the uterus, vagina and bladder, dysentery, enlarged anal glands, obesity, dropsy, a strong dose dissolves stones in the bladder.

Human Dose - 2 to 4mls of tincture 3 times a day.

Caution - If used over a long period it may decrease vitamin B1.

Hypericum (St Johns Wort)

Actions - Anti-inflammatory, astringent, anti-viral, anti-spasmodic, nervine, vulnerary, antibacterial.

The name St Johns Wort came from the Knights of St John of Jerusalem who used the herb to treat battle wounds.

Uses - Taken internally has a sedative and pain reducing effect, neuralgic pain, anxiety, tension, rheumatic pain, sciatica, for pains that shoot along the nerves, as a lotion it will speed the healing of wounds and bruises and is used where there is damage to the nerve rich areas, varicose veins and mild burns. Good for inflamed joints and rheumatic pain. In humans recently the herb has become popular to use as an antidepressant especially for cases of anxiety. Use as a lotion on wounds especially in the nerve rich areas such as the lips and fingers. As a lotion it is commonly mixed with Calendula, Homoeopaths call this lotion Hypercal.

Cats and Dogs - Excellent wound herb and good for all nerve injuries. Good for highly strung, hysterical cats and dogs or those who have suffered some emotional or physical trauma.

Human Dose - 1 to 4mls of tincture 3 times a day.

Caution - Animals that overdose on Hypericum become photosensitive and have to be locked in the barn for a while so as not to become sun burnt.

Hyssop

Actions - Anti spasmodic, expectorant, antiviral, nervine, diaphoretic, sedative, carminative.

A important plant in pectoral complaints because it removes mucous accumulations and also tones up the membranes and fortifies the whole system along with being a respiratory antiviral. Is a mild vermifuge the Nordic countries use it as a vermifuge for delicate lambs and kids. Coughs, bronchitis, chronic catarrh, colds and flu's, anxiety states, hysteria, petit mal.

Uses - Treatment of cough especially the more spasmodic coughs such as whooping, sore throat, pneumonia, pleurisy, TB, or any respiratory disease, worms, eye disorders, conjunctivitis.

Human Dose - 1 to 4mls 3 times a day.

Juniper

Actions - Diuretic, antiseptic, carminative, anti-rheumatic.

The whole plant is a tonic and nerve stimulant, excellent anti-septic in conditions like cystitis, stimulating to the kidney nephrons (avoid in kidney disease), the bitter action aids digestion and eases flatulent colic.

Uses - Treatment of inflamed liver and kidneys, gallstones, jaundice, obesity, sciatica, rheumatism, blood ailments, acid milk, malaria.

Human Dose - 0.5 to 1mls of tincture 3 times a day.

Caution - Avoid in kidney disease. Avoid in pregnancy.

Kelp

Actions – Anti-hypothyroid, anti-rheumatic, nutritive,

Used mainly for under active thyroid (iodine) especially when it is thought to be the cause of overweight. Helps in the relief of rheumatism internally and externally. Added to feed for nutrition. Can be used to slim fat horses. Make sure that iodine isn't in any of the supplements you are already giving. It is good for coat and hoof conditions.

Horses - 2 tablespoons a day for overweight horses half the amount for normal.

Ladys Mantle

Actions - Astringent, diuretic, anti-inflammatory, emmenagogue, vulnerary.

This herb has an affinity to the womb where it helps with pain, bleeding and getting the cycle back to normal. Horses, goats and sheep seek out the herb, the plant is tonic and an important fortifier for the blood and walls of the arteries, it is a old herbal remedy for diabetes, reduces period pains and excessive bleeding, diarrhea, sores, ulcers a good menopause herb.

Cats and Dogs - A good female herb for abdominal ailments, injuries after delivery or damage and debility, to strengthen the developing foetus in the womb, for inclination to miscarry and prolapse of the uterus.

Uses - Treatment for lack of appetite, wasting, weak blood, sluggish blood, all weaknesses of the arteries, heart disease, taken from one period to another it is reputed to aid conception in barren animals.

Human Dose - 2 to 4mls of tincture 3 times daily.

Lemon Balm (Melissa)

Actions - Carminative, antispasmodic, anti-depressive, diaphoretic, hypotensive, emmenagogue, nervine, rejunative tonic, Anti-viral.

In the past this plant was used to attract bees by rubbing it all around a new hive and the smell made the bees want to stay. The name Melissa is Greek for honey bee. The Arabs say it gives intelligence to any animal that feeds upon it.

Relieves spasms in the digestive tract and is used in

flatulent dyspepsia. Good for digestive problems brought on from worry, anxiety and stress. Has a tonic effect on the heart and circulatory system causing mild vasodilatation of the peripheral blood vessels which can help to lower blood pressure and also may calm the electrical activity of the heart. Has also been used in animals for a retained afterbirth and as a anti-viral for infections such as herpes.

Horses - 1 cup full of dried herb twice daily.

Caution - Can sometimes lower thyroid function.

Licorice

Actions - Expectorant, demulcent, anti-inflammatory, adrenal agent, anti-spasmodic, mild laxative.

The root part is used , possessing unique pectoral and emollient properties, it is also nutritive and slightly laxative, It contains the building blocks of hormones, has a marked effect on the endocrine system, catarrh, gastric and peptic ulcers, abdominal colic. Its ability to soothe irritated mucous membranes and to break up phlegm and ease coughing sees licorice employed in respiratory conditions, coughing, bronchitis, and chest colds. Can be used for treating inflammatory and allergic conditions. Licorice has effects on the adrenal glands which are protective, restorative, tonic and stimulatory. These properties can aid the horse which is recovering from steroid therapy or abuse.

Uses - Treatment of cough, inflamed throat,

pneumonia, pleurisy, TB, all catarrhal conditions, gallstones, chronic constipation, mild worms in young animals, female infertility, pains of colic.

Human Dose - Tincture 2 to 6mls of tincture 3 times daily.

Horses - 1 teaspoon full of powder daily.

Caution - Do not use with high blood pressure. Long term use depletes potassium which raises the blood pressure. Don't use with steroids.

Lime Blossom (Linden)

Actions - Nervine, antispasmodic, diaphoretic, diuretic, mild astringent.

Possesses powerful nervine and blood cleansing properties, used for fits and nervous twitching of all kinds including epilepsy, a good tonic for bees, nervous tension, as a prophylactic against arteriosclerosis, migraines, feverish colds and flu.

Uses - Treatment of all nervous ailments especially epilepsy, twitching, vertigo, good for colds and to remove the slime and mucous from the system, treatment of vomiting, heart pains, fevers, treatment of tumors by poultice.

Human Dose - 1 to 2mls of tincture 3 times a day.

Marsh Mallow

Actions - Demulcent, anti-inflammatory, expectorant, astringent.

Its therapeutic effects are largely due to its significant mucilage and pectin content, aided by its anti-inflammatory properties. The foliage of the mallow is eaten by all animals, the roots are the main part used for internal medicine and also the leaves which are especially used for inflammation of the stomach and bowel and especially used for ulcers, it contains over half its weight in sweet tasting mucilage which has unique properties of lubricating, soothing and healing. A poultice can be used for all inflammatory conditions. Horses who have colic, or who are scouring, can benefit from the soothing and healing effects of marshmallow also see Slippery Elm. Consider using as a supplement for horses prone to colic and ulcers. Marshmallow can also be used to soothe inflamed and irritated mucous membranes of the respiratory and urinary systems. Dry coughs, sore throats, urinary tract inflammation and cystitis have all been relieved by the effects of marshmallow.

Uses - Treatment of sore throats, pulmonary catarrhs, pleurisy, cystitis, diarrhea, dysentery, ulcers, bowel inflammations and hemorrhages.

Externally - All skin eruptions, abrasions, swellings, inflammations, bruises, sore inflamed udders.

Human Dose - 2 to 4mls of tincture 3 times a day.

Horses - 1 to 2 hands full infused. Give 1 cup twice a day. 2 tablespoons of the powdered root 2 to 3 times daily.

Marigold see Calendula

Meadowsweet

Actions - Anti-inflammatory, anti-rheumatic, antacid, anti-emetic, stomachic, astringent.

A important fever and diarrhea herb, the gypsies use as a spring tonic for their animals, eaten plentifully by goats and sheep, acts to protect and soothe the mucous membranes of the digestive tract reducing excess acidity and easing nausea, heart burn, hyperacidity, gastritis, peptic ulcers. This herb is a good acid balancer and is good for correcting over acid systems. Meadowsweet is the forerunner of aspirin as this is the first herb it was synthesized from in 1835 but as this herb contains its own buffering agents it is gentle on the stomach. Used to help reduce inflammation and for pain relief in case of arthritic conditions. Useful alone or in combination with other herbs for effective pain management.

Uses - Fevers, arthritis, diarrhea and the above mentioned.

Human Dose - 1 to 4mls of tincture 3 times daily.

Horses - 1 cup full of dried flowers twice daily.

Caution - Avoid if sensitive to salicylates. Not for Cats as they don't like the Aspirin part of this herb.

Mistletoe

Actions - Nervine, hypotensive, cardiac depressant,

possibly anti-tumor.

It will quiet soothe and tone the nervous system, acts directly on the vagus nerve to reduce heart rate while strengthening the walls of the peripheral capillaries, reduces blood pressure and eases arteriosclerosis, nervous tachycardia, headache due to high blood pressure.

Uses - Treatment of nervous ailments, epilepsy, hysteria, heart tonic, uterine and vaginal bleeding.

Human Dose - 1 to 4mls of tincture 3 times a day.

Milk Thistle

Actions - Cholagogue, galactagogue, demulcent.

This herb is said to rejuvenate the liver, for problems like hepatitis it is used alone at first as it drains the liver probably by its action of stimulating the gallbladder to release bile. Much of the therapeutic benefit of the seeds is attributed to a group of potent antioxidant bioflavonoids, known together as silymarin, which are able to guard and stabilize cell membranes, preventing the invasion of toxins, as well as enhance the regeneration of liver cells already damaged by detoxification processes. for horses who have suffered liver damage from poisons, infections, high worm burdens, reactions to worming drugs, or excessive drug use. Can be taken long term and needs be taken for a prolonged period at least 4-12 weeks to be of most benefit In disease like hepatitis you just use it by itself sometimes for months after this time you can consider adding Dandelion.

Used to increase milk production in mothers and for gallbladder problems.

Uses - Liver problems, gallbladder problems, hepatitis, to increase milk production.

Human Dose - 1 to 2mls of tincture 3 times daily.

Dose - 1 tablespoon of seed given morning and night. Good for long term treatment.

Milk Thistle and Dandelion Together

Actions of Milk Thistle - Cholagogue, galactagogue, demulcent. Known as the liver regenerator.

Milk Thistle and dandelion together make a good and gentle liver cleanser, detoxifier and repairer. Use for liver or kidney damage, hepatitis (include Echinacea), jaundice, leptospirosis and parvo virus recovery. It may be helpful in chronic skin disorders, tumors and cancer. This is a major antioxidant. Pets that have been on a lot of veterinary drugs, heart worm prevention, vaccinations, de-worming drugs or chemotherapy need this healing from these herbs.

Human Dose - Is 1 to 2mls of tincture 3 times daily.

Motherwort

Actions - Sedative, emmenagogue, antispasmodic,

cardiac tonic.

As its species name indicates, it has long been considered a nerve and heart remedy. It strengthens heart function, particularly where it is weak. Antispasmodic and sedative, the herb causes relaxation rather than drowsiness. Motherwort is considered a life giving plant, beneficial for all female disorders and a general heart tonic. Delayed or suppressed menses especially where anxiety or tension are involved, specific for over rapid heartbeat brought on by anxiety or tension, lowers high blood pressure and is used for the pains of birth and given for a few days after so as to prevent bleeding and infection.

Human Dose - 1 to 4mls of tincture 3 times daily.

Horses - 1 cup full of the leaf given daily.

Mullein

Actions - Expectorant, demulcent, mild diuretic, mild sedative, vulnerary.

The herb is famed for its powers in pulmonary ailments being much used in lung ailments of cattle, a bone flesh and cartilage builder, aids in healing respiratory ailments, asthma, bronchitis, sinus congestion, soothing to any inflammation and relieves pain, acts to relieve spasms and clears the lungs, tones mucous membranes of the respiratory system, inflammation of the trachea, painful coughs. The leaves of Mullein were traditionally fed to animals that cough especially horses.

Uses - Coughs, pneumonia, bronchitis, pleurisy, TB, asthma, diarrhea, internal bleeding of the lung and bowel.

Human Dose - 1 to 4mls of tincture 3 times a day.

Horse - 1 cup full of herb daily added to feed.

Myrrh

Actions - Anti microbial, astringent, carminative, anti-catarrhal, expectorant, vulnerary, antiseptic, antifungal, alterative.

Stimulates production of white blood cells and also has a good anti-microbial action so this is a good herb for immune boosting and fighting diseases.

Uses - Stomach viruses, coughs, asthma, infections of the mouth, mouth ulcers, gingivitis, sinusitis, laryngitis.

Externally - Healing and antiseptic to wounds and abrasions.

Human Dose - 1 to 4mls 3 times a day.

Cautions - Use only in small amounts for short periods. Large amounts can speed heartbeat.

Nasturtium

Actions - Anti microbial, expectorant, anthelmintic.

The plant has a hot biting character especially in the seeds which were once used to make a popular pickle. Animals eat the whole plant greedily. The seeds of this plant are collected and used on poultry as a wormer. The seeds can be preserved in vinegar and used as a tonic and anti-worm remedy. A powerful anti-microbial especially when used locally on bacterial infections. Internally use for infections more so in the respiratory system such as bronchitis, flu and colds where it is used in breaking up congestion in the respiratory passages.

Uses - Bacterial infections, respiratory infections, as a tonic, poor sight, worms. Locally as a general antiseptic.

Human Dosage - 1 to 4mls of tincture 3 times daily. For animals several handfuls of leaves fed daily. For worms 1 dessertspoon of seeds (the smaller the animal decrease the dose).

Neem

Actions - Anti-inflammatory, alterative, antibacterial, antiviral, antifungal, anthelmintic, bitter tonic, immune stimulant.

The name in Sanskrit means curer of all ailments and another name it is called is village pharmacy. Its antibacterial properties are good for Staph and Clostridia, Neem effectively kills lice and is good for topical applications to skin problems.

Uses - Ring worm, eczema , rash, arthritis and rheumatism and is used for malaria. Use as a wash for ticks, mites, scabies and fleas.

Cautions - Not for use for infants and the elderly

and not for long term internal use.

Nettles

Actions - Astringent, diuretic, galactagogue, tonic, nutritive.

Nettle is perhaps best known as a highly nutritious feed herb/fodder for animals, and has been used through the ages for this purpose. It is considered a spring tonic and detoxifier for human and animal alike. One of the richest sources of chlorophyll in the vegetable kingdom, rich in iron, lime, sodium, Vit C, chlorine and contains much protein. Preventative against many ailments, increases milk yield, fattener for poultry. Good astringent for stopping bleeding anywhere but especially in the urinary tract. Good for eczema in the young especially in the nervous young. Good for pregnant and nursing mothers. The seeds can be used as a thyroid tonic.

Uses - Treatment of wasting diseases, poor appetite, lung disorders, blood impurities, worms, fever, cold, hay fever, allergies, eczema, diarrhea, hemorrhage.

Externally - Paralysis, rheumatism, arthritis, loss of muscular power.

Human Dose - 1 to 4mls of tincture 3 times a day.

Horse - 1 cup full of herb 2 to 3 times daily.

Caution - Only buy the product prepared for herbal use.

Oats

Actions - Nerve tonic, anti-depressant, nutritive, demulcent, vulnerary.

Oats are a strength giving cereal low in starch high in mineral content especially potassium, phosphorus, magnesium and calcium and also the B vitamins. Is a nerve tonic and bone builder used for nervous debility, nervous exhaustion, general debility, skin conditions.

Uses - As a nutritive food, remedy and cure for rickets, important for strong teeth, hooves, horns, nails and hair.

Human Dose - 1 to 2mls of tincture 3 times a day.

Parsley

Actions - Diuretic, carminative, emmenagogue, expectorant.

Well-liked by sheep and goats, improves their milk yield and keeps them free from foot ills. It is a great enricher of the blood being very rich in iron and copper. Nutrient, digestive tract tonic, diuretic, high in potassium minerals and vitamins, bladder and kidney infections, incontinence, blood cleanser, immune builder, tonic for the blood vessels, aids in afterbirth pains, mainly used as a diuretic, carminative and emmenagogue. Is a good source of chlorophyll, parsley is useful for combating bad breath. Its diuretic properties are beneficial in: arthritic/rheumatic conditions associated with poor kidney function; urinary infections; kidney and bladder stones. Parsley also acts as a digestive tonic by easing spasms and minimizing flatulence.

Uses - Treatment of all disorders of the kidneys and bladder, gravel, stones, congestion, cystitis, jaundice, obesity, dropsy, worms, rheumatism, prostrate problems, sciatica, swellings of the joints, the root can be used for constipation and obstructions of the intestines.

Human Dose - 2 to 4mls of tincture 3 times daily

Horse - 1 cup of dried herb twice daily.

Dogs: - Use larger amounts of parsley tea – 1- 2 tablespoon 3/4 times daily.

Can also add finely chopped parsley into their daily meals once or twice a week to help keep kidneys cleansed and free of disease.

Caution - Do not use in pregnancy.

Passion Flower

Actions - Sedative, antispasmodic, anodyne, relaxant, epilepsy, shingles, asthma, hypotensive.

A good herb for insomnia and a very effective herb for nerve pains especially in conditions like shingles. This herbs focus is more on restlessness and irritability, hysteria and anxiety and is soothing to the mentally worried and overworked it acts on nervousness especially due to unrest, agitation, worry, exhaustion and cerebral excitement. Can be of benefit to horses that are generally nervous and apprehensive. Used in the treatment of convulsions, epilepsy, tremors, hypertension, nervous breakdowns, migraines and neuralgias.

Human Doses - Tincture 1 to 4mls of tincture 3 times daily, 1 teaspoon of dried herb in tea 3 times daily.

Horse - 2 teaspoons of powdered herb daily or half a cup of herb daily.

Cautions - Large doses may cause nausea and vomiting. Do not use while pregnant.

Pau D'Arco

Actions - Alterative, anodyne, analgesic, antifungal, antibacterial, anti-inflammatory, antioxidant, antiviral, diuretic, immune stimulant.

This herb comes from Brazil and is used by the Indians there. It possesses properties that are antibiotic, tumor inhibiting, virus killing, anti-fungal and anti-malarial. Builds up the immune system. Its anti-inflammatory action applies especially in the stomach and intestines as well as for conditions such as cystitis, inflammation of the cervix, arthritis and prostatitis; it is a good herb for fighting fungal infections while building up the immune system. This herb is used for lung, colon and prostate cancer. It contains a chemical called lapachol that inhibits tumor cell growth by preventing them from metabolizing oxygen. Pau D'Arco also lowers blood sugar levels and acts as a mild laxative.

Human Dose - 3 to 5mls of tincture 3 times a day.

Horse- 1 to 2 teaspoons of powdered herb daily.

Pennyroyal

Actions - Carminative, diaphoretic, stimulant, emmenagogue, insecticide.

The forerunner of the cultivated mints, animals seek it for its tonic and stimulating properties, herdsmen use it after calving as a stimulant and restorative to the cow, abdominal colic due to wind, spasmodic pain, eases anxiety, its main use is as a emmenagogue to stimulate the menstrual process and strengthen uterine contractions. Helpful against nausea and nervous conditions.

Uses - Treatment of digestive ailments including failing appetite, sour stomach and internal gas, cough, pneumonia, fever, bronchitis and pleurisy, after birth exhaustion, female complaints.

Externally used as a insect repellant (oil) and a lotion for itching skin eg rashes, psoriasis etc.

Human Dose - 1 to 2mls of tincture 3 times daily.

Caution - Do not use in pregnancy or in large doses.

Peppermint

Actions - Carminative, diaphoretic, anti-spasmodic, anti-emetic, nervine, analgesic, anti-septic.

Best known for its ability to aid digestion and relieve gastrointestinal distress. Peppermint owes most of its medicinal value to menthol, which is cooling, anesthetic, antiseptic and soothing to the stomach. For horses, peppermint's aroma is useful for tempting fussy eaters and/or helping to mask the smell of less pleasant herbs in their feed. It eases flatulence/bloating, increases the flow of bile from the liver and relaxes both gastrointestinal spasms and tight skeletal muscles.

Uses- Nausea, heartburn, indigestion, colic, flatulence, dyspepsia, vomiting, fevers, migraine headaches and irritable bowel syndrome (IBS) and for travel sickness think of adding Ginger for this.

Human Dose - 1 to 2mls of tincture 3 times a day.

Horse - 1 to 2 cups of dried herb daily.

Caution - May reduce milk flow if breast feeding.

Plantain

Actions - Expectorant, demulcent, astringent, antibacterial, diuretic.

Goats and sheep enjoy its foliage and poultry seek out the seeds. Plantain clears heat and removes excess fluid from the body while at the same time soothing inflammation and irritated tissues. The whole plant yields a soothing mucilage similar to linseed, gentle expectorant while soothing sore and inflamed membranes, coughs, bronchitis etc. Its astringency aids in diarrhea and cystitis where there is bleeding. Is good for using in the treatment of stomach ulcers and has been used for blood poisoning. The plant is high in chlorophyll and good for use on wounds.

Cats and Dogs - Plantain is used for the entire range of diseases of the respiratory organs, particularly congested lungs, bronchial asthma and TB. It purifies the blood, lungs and stomach and is good for bad blood, kidney disorders, eczema, herpes and coughs. It helps convalescents especially when they need to gain weight. Also used in liver and bladder diseases.

Uses - Treatment of dysentery, hemorrhages, internal obstructions and ulcers, fevers.

Externally - Wounds, sores, ulcers and all bites, eye disorders.

Human Dose - 2 to 3mls of tincture 3 times a day.

Poke Root - Phytolacca

Actions - Purgative, emetic, stimulant, anti-rheumatic and anti-catarrhal.

May be seen primarily as a remedy for use in infections of the upper respiratory tract removing catarrh and aiding in the cleansing of the lymphatic glands, it may be used for catarrh, tonsillitis, laryngitis and swollen glands. It will be found to be of value to problems elsewhere in the body involving the lymphatic system especially mastitis (Homoeopathic form works faster). Also used in long standing cases of rheumatism. Poke Root stimulates the immune system by increasing T cell activity. Care must be taken with this herb as in large doses it is a powerful emetic and purgative. Can be used as a lotion in mastitis. This herb in the past has been known as cancer root and has been used for breast cancer and tumors.

Uses - Mastitis and other lymphatic problems.

External Use - Breast cancer, tumors, mastitis, boils, fungal infections, shingles, psoriasis, scabies and eczema.

Human Dose - Half to 1ml up to of tincture 3 times daily.

Cautions - This is a very strong herb so use it very carefully in small doses.

Raspberry

Actions - Astringent, tonic, refrigerant, parturient.

Raspberry leaf has been used for mares with oestrus problems and the attendant behavioral disturbances. For mares that have had or may have difficulty conceiving it can be given for a period prior to mating. Generally, raspberry leaf is used to tone the uterine muscles, encourage an easy labor, and hemorrhaging during and after birth

Highly tonic and cleansing improving the condition of the organism during pregnancy ensuring speedy and strong expulsion of the fetus at birth, use as a drench in retained afterbirth, acclaimed as a tonic for male animals and as a cure for sterility, becomes especially potent for female use when blended with feverfew - 3 parts to 1 part of feverfew. As a astringent it can be used in diarrhea and leucorrhoea, it is valuable in easing mouth problems such as mouth ulcers, bleeding gums and inflammations

Uses - Prevention and treatment of all female ailments, retained afterbirth, digestive ailments including diarrhea, treatment of mouth and throat ailments as a gargle.

Human Dose - 2 to 4mls of tincture 3 times daily.

Horse - 1 cup full daily.

Red Clover

Actions - Alterative, diuretic, expectorant, antispasmodic, nutritive.

The flowers are a powerful tonic and a cure for nervous twitches, wasting bodies and cough. The whole plant is sedative. Good for treating conditions like eczema and psoriasis and other chronic skin conditions. In the respiratory system we can use the actions of expectorant and antispasmodic to treat conditions such as bronchitis, whooping cough and maybe the eczema and asthma syndrome and as this herb seems to have a affinity for the throat we could use it for tonsillitis to. In the nervous system we can use the antispasmodic action to treat stress and nervousness along with hypertension. The alterative action of this herb helps to clean out the body and makes this herbs action on the skin very effective and it is probably this action that makes it useful in cancers especially breast and Ovary cancer. The herb has proved beneficial in cancers of the stomach and throat. This herb is in a lot of female formulas now because they extract the Isoflavones (Plant Hormones) from it and it is said to be very rich in these.

Uses - Tonic, treatment for general debility, weak nerves, throat ailments, cancers, tumors, detox, skin diseases and respiratory problems.

Doses - Tincture 2 to 6mls of tincture 3 times a day. 1 to 3 teaspoon full of dried herb in tea 3 times a day.

Rose Hips

Actions - Nutrient, mild laxative, mild diuretic, mild astringent.

The foliage is enjoyed by all animals. The flowers are tonic and astringent. The fruits are slightly aperient and rich in vitamin C. A good spring tonic and aid to general debility and exhaustion. Used to fight infection and curb stress. Rosehips are often fed to horses recuperating from injury as they help to restore the immune system and aid tissue repair and leaking capillaries with their bioflavonoids.

Human Dose - 2 to 4mls of tincture three time daily.

Horse - 1 cup full of infusion twice daily.

Rosemary

Actions - Carminative, aromatic, antispasmodic, anti-depressive, antiseptic, parasiticide.

It imparts a fine fragrance and tonic properties to the milk of goat and sheep which graze it eagerly. The powdered form is used on wounds as a antiseptic, nerve tonic, carminative, insecticide, acts as a circulatory and nerve stimulant, headache.

Uses - Treatment of all ailments of the heart, rheumatism, fits, epilepsy, paralysis, gastritis, diarrhea, dysentery.

Externally - Wounds, falling hair and nervous spasms.

Human Dose - 1 to 2mls 3 times a day.

Caution - Excessive large doses can poison and cause death.

Rue

Actions - Antispasmodic, emmenagogue, anti tussive, abortifacient.

The essential principal of the plant is Rutin which possesses most potent powers strengthening weakened blood vessels, toning the nerves and glands and imparting hardness to bones teeth and nails, highly antiseptic and is also a insecticide, it is also an old remedy for the prevention and cure of rabies. Regulates menses, used to bring on suppressed menses, the anti-spasmodic action is used to relax smooth muscles especially in the digestive system where it will ease gripping and bowel tension, spasmodic coughs, lowers elevated blood pressure.

Uses - Treatment of fevers, epilepsy, neuralgia, heart disease, ailments of the arteries and veins, worms, all skin parasites including scabies and ringworm,.

Human Dose - 1 to 4mls of tincture avoid in pregnancy.

Caution - Avoid in pregnancy.

Reshi Mushroom

Actions - Immune stimulant, antibacterial, anti-tumor, adaptogen, rejuvenative, anti-inflammatory

As a immune stimulant it helps to activate the phagocytosis of macrophages and may increase interferon. Aids in the prevention of illness as well as in recovery. Helps normalize blood pressure reduces cholesterol and can inhibit histamine release. Inhibits the inflammation associated with allergies, bronchitis, conjunctivitis and rheumatism. Good for treating chronic hepatitis. Good for over overcoming fatigue, anxiety and stress while improving stamina at the same time.

Uses - Good as an all round immune booster and restorative tonic. Works well with its fellow mushroom Shitake as they tend to complement each others actions and together they can be used to attack acute viral diseases. In chronic disease use 1/10 of the recommended dose.

Shitake Mushroom

Actions - Immune stimulant, antiviral, rejuvinative, aphrodisiac.

Animal studies have shown an antiviral and anti tumour activity as well as the stimulation of killer T cells. Shitake enhances the stem cells in the bone marrow to create more B and T cells. Lowers blood pressure by helping the body get rid of excessive salt and can be used in AIDs like diseases. Stimulates the production of interferon and provides significant protection against type A Viruses which causes epidemic influenza.

Uses - Good as an all-round immune booster and restorative tonic. Works well with its fellow mushroom Reshi as they tend to complement each others actions and together they can be used to attack acute viral diseases. In chronic disease use 1/10 of the recommended dose.

Sage

Actions - Carminative, antispasmodic, antiseptic, astringent.

Sage is well liked by animals and as with other aromatics makes the milk refreshing, tonic and increases the milk yield, it is a nervine, digestive and blood cleanser, a first rate remedy for all disorders of the throat, lungs and ears, inflamed and bleeding gums, inflamed tongue or general mouth inflammation, mouth ulcers, a good mouth wash.

Uses - Treatment of nerve debility, paralysis, all gastric ailments, constipation, obesity and female ailments, eczema, fevers, wound infections.

Human Dose - 2 to 4mls of tincture 3 times a day. For sore mouths and throat ailments give mixed with honey.

Horse - Infuse 1 teaspoon of powdered herb in 2 cups of water. Use in small doses. For sore mouths and throat ailments give mixed with honey.

Cats and Dogs - For inflammations of the mouth, throat and tonsils.

Caution - Stimulates the muscles of the uterus so should be avoided during pregnancy.

Sarsaparilla

Actions - Alterative, diuretic, diaphoretic, anti-rheumatic, tonic.

Has a purifying effect on the genito urinary tract helping in the clearing of infections and the excretion of uric acid. Has chemicals and properties that aid in the production of testosterone, eliminates poisons and toxins from the blood and helps clean the system, useful in scaling skin conditions such as psoriasis, used in rheumatism and arthritis.

Uses - Rheumatism, arthritis, gout, skin eruptions, ringworm, internal inflammations, colds, catarrh.

Human Dose - 1 to 2mls of tincture 3 times a day.

Slippery Elm Bark Powder

Actions - Demulcent, emollient, nutrient, astringent.

Slippery elm bark provides a nutritious gruel which

also possesses remarkable medicinal properties acting as a poultice both internally and externally. A nutrient and food for very old or young or weak especially if mixed with honey, coats and heals all inflamed tissues internally and externally and is used for the stomach, intestines, ulcers, ulcerative colitis, enteritis, dysentery, constipation and internal bleeding of the digestive tract.

Uses - Treatment of all digestive complaints especially ulcers for which it is a specific, dysentery, all pectoral disorders including TB, lung and bronchial hemorrhage, wasting diseases, rickets, stunted growth. Calves with scour can be kept alive on this mixed with honey while the non-treated can die.

Externally - A poultice for all skin ailments especially old ailments and hard swellings.

Human Dose - 1 part powder to 8 parts water. Animals - 2 tablespoons mixed into a smooth texture with 1 tablespoon of honey.

Horse - Mix 2 tablespoons of powder with honey to form a paste and dose orally or blend with a cup of water.

Shepherds Purse

Actions - Uterine stimulant, astringent, diuretic.

Possesses important astringent properties, all animals like this herb and poultry seek it eagerly.

A gentle diuretic, diarrhea, wounds, reduces

excessive menstruation.

Uses - Treatment of hemorrhages internal and external, profuse bleeding of deep wounds, kidney ailments, female problems.

Human Dose - 1 to 2mls of tincture 3 times a day.

Skullcap

Actions - Nervine tonic, sedative, antispasmodic.

Supreme nerve herb and has restored many cases of nervous disorders, nervous tension, seizures, epilepsy, PMS, carminative nervine and nervous system repairer, pain reliever, spinal problems, twitching muscles, rheumatism, high blood pressure, restlessness, nervous heart conditions.

Uses - Treatment of all nervous complaints especially hysteria, fits, meningitis, nervous spasms, gastroenteritis, an old cure for rabies.

Human Dose - 2 to 4mls of tincture 3 times daily.

St Johns Wort see Hypericum

Sweet Violets

Actions - Alterative, expectorant, anti-inflammatory, anti-cancer, diuretic, antifungal, antiseptic.

Is used with Red Clover as a detoxifier and a blood cleanser. Especially useful to animals that have had a toxic reaction to Vaccination. Good for coughs and bronchitis. Can be used as a poultice on cancer tumors.

Uses - Skin problems, tumors, warts, behavior reactions or other aggravations from vaccination, digestive disorders, seizures, cancer, cysts, boils, abscesses, chronic skin diseases.

Human Dose - 1 to 2mls 3 times daily.

Senna Pods

Actions - Cathartic

One of the most important laxatives because it is also a cleanser and restorative of the entire digestive system. The griping tendency is diminished by the addition of powdered ginger. As heat destroy the properties of this herb it should be prepared as a cold water infusion steeping the pods or leaves for a minimum of 4 hours.

Uses - Treatment of constipation.

Dose - Five large senna pods for an average dog, 7 for sheep, 8 for goats 20 for horses and 24 for cows. Soak in cold water for a minimum of 4 hours but preferably 7 hours. A half cup fill of water for 6 pods, 3/4 cup for 10 pods, one and a half cups for 20 and 24. Add a pinch of ginger to 6 to 10 pods and half a teaspoon to 20 to 24. Give the dose last thing at night at least 2 hours after food has been taken.

Tansy

Actions - Digestive bitter, carminative, emmenagogue, vermifuge, anthelmintic.

Cows and sheep eat the herb, powerful worm expellant, effective against round worm and thread worm and may be used in children as a enema, as a bitter it will stimulate the digestive process, eases dyspepsia, stimulate menses.

Uses - Treatment of all types of worms, debility, causes abortion.

Human Dose - 1 to 2mls of tincture 3 time a day.

Caution - Avoid during Pregnancy.

Tea Tree Oil

Australian Tea Tree Oil is one of the world's best antiseptics and is also anti-bacterial, anti-fungal and anti-viral which means you can use it with good results on virtually any wound on the skin.

Use for external applications.

Thyme

Actions - Carminative, antimicrobial, antispasmodic, expectorant, astringent, anthelmintic.

Eaten by sheep and goats and is a milk tonic for them, the whole herb is tonic and antiseptic, A favourite Bee herb and should be planted by all apiaries, can be used for digestive or respiratory infections, use as a gargle for laryngitis or tonsillitis, eases sore throats and coughs, bronchitis, whooping cough, asthma, diarrhea and dyspepsia and sluggish digestion,

Uses - Treatment of all digestive complaints including colic, inflammation of the liver, rickets, all pectoral ailments, hysteria, nervousness, sciatica, retention of afterbirth, inflamed or diseased uterus, metritis, worms including hook worm.

Human Dose - 2 to 4mls of tincture 3 times a day.

Valerian

Actions - Sedative, antispasmodic, hypnotic, hypotensive, carminative.

A powerful nervine and sedative stronger than other herbal sedatives, pain reliever, reduces anxiety, hysteria, soothes the nervous system, reduces high blood pressure, slows and strengthens the heart and calms palpitations, useful for muscle spasms, arthritic pain, spinal injuries, aids indigestion and gas, insomnia, cramps, colic, can help with migraines. Valerian root is one of the most widely used herbal nervines for calming horses as it can relieve anxiety and excitability without reducing the horse's mental faculties or their physical ability to perform.

Uses - Treatment of epilepsy, hysteria, acute constipation, worms, malaria, pain and for sensitive nervous animals.

Externally - The oil is used as a rub for paralyzed limbs, cramps, swollen arteries and veins.

Human Dose - 2 to 4mls of tincture 3 times a day.

Horse - 1 to 2 tablespoons twice daily. Give more for a pain killing action.

Caution - Do not mix with drug tranquillizers.

Vervain

Actions - Nerve tonic, hepatic, sedative, antispasmodic, diaphoretic.

A favorite of Hippocrates, valuable in every type of fever use in the early stages, nervous disorders, eye problems, plague remedy of ancient times, strengthens the nervous system while relaxing any tension or stress, depression especially if it comes on after an illness, seizures, hysteria, inflammation of the gallbladder, jaundice, use as a mouth wash in gum disease.

Uses - Treatments of all fevers, fits, convulsions, hysteria, liver complaints, gallstones.

Externally - Weak and inflamed eyes, inflamed throats, sore and ulcerated mouths.

Human Dose - 2 to 4mls of tincture 3 times a day.

Wild Yam

Actions - Antispasmodic, anti-inflammatory, anti-rheumatic,

The first birth control pills were once based on this remedy. Used for severe digestive pain in conditions such as colic, dysmenorrhea, and ovarian and uterine pains. Also used in the treatment of rheumatoid arthritis especially when there is painful inflammation. Muscle cramps and spasms, nerve pains and threatened miscarriage.

Human Dose - 2 to 4mls of tincture 3 times a day.

Horse - 1 tablespoon of powder twice daily.

Willow Bark (White Willow)

Actions - Febrifuge, bitter tonic, astringent, antiseptic, analgesic, anti-inflammatory, anti-rheumatic.

Willow Bark can be thought of as caveman's Aspirin as it was developed from this. Cattle and horses eat the young shoots and foliage. It is a refrigerant herb valuable in fevers and pain relief but can take a while to get into the system so think of looking for results especially in pain in about a day's time.

Uses - Treatment of all fevers, debility, enteritis, colic, pleurisy, rheumatism, sciatica and urinary infections as the excretion of salicylic acid in urine soothes a inflamed tract.

Externally - Rickets and cramp.

Human Dose - 2 to 4mls of tincture 3 times a day.

Horse - 2 teaspoonful's of powdered bark twice daily. Externally - Use the same brew as a massage in pain effected areas.

Witch Hazel

Actions - Astringent one of the most widely used

ones. Antiseptic.

As with all astringents this herb may be used wherever there is bleeding both externally and internally, commonly used for piles, bruises and inflamed swellings, varicose veins, diarrhea.

Uses - Internally to heal ulcerated and burnt tissues in cases of poisoning, stomach and intestinal ulcers, Externally - wounds, sores, bruises, ulcers, inflammation of the organs of reproduction, torn udders resulting in milk leakage, inflamed udders and glands, sore eyes and inflamed ears.

Human Dose - 1 to 2 mls of tincture 3 times daily.

Withania (Ashwagandha)

Actions - Adaptogen, analgesic, anti-tumor, hormone regulator, pregnancy tonic, rejuvinative.

This herb is a pregnancy tonic for both the foetus and a weak mother, relieves pain by lowering serotonin levels which contribute to the sensitivity of pain receptors in the body. Good for debility, nervous exhaustion especially due to stress and chronic diseases especially those marked by inflammation. Retards various aspects of the aging process and increases stamina and also sexual desire.

Doses - As on packet.

Wood Betony

Actions - Alterative, analgesic, antispasmodic,

astringent, Bitter tonic, sedative, circulatory stimulant, diuretic.

Juliette de Bairacli Levy says the whole plant possesses a pungent and peculiar aroma especially when trampled on. This would show the plant to have a high oil content. Was once used as a smoke and snuff to treat headaches. Wood Betony is used for severe pains in the face and head consider it for horses with severe sinus or those who always toss there head.

Uses - Treatment of debility, gastritis, diarrhea, acidity, glandular deficiency, arthritis, rheumatism, exhaustion, sciatica, hypertension, kidney dysfunction.

Externally - arthritis, rheumatism, sciatica, rickets, tumors, swellings, boils, abscesses, corns, warts and blisters, gingivitis, as a poultice to draw out splinters and boils.

Horse - 2 handfuls made into a syrup by simmering in 1 and a half pints of water to which has been added a quarter pound of brown sugar or half a cup full of the dried herb twice daily.

Wormwood

Actions - Bitter tonic, carminative, anthelmintic, anti-inflammatory.

The foliage is eaten by horses, cows and sheep. Its chief merits are worm expellant (round worm and pinworm) and tonic. A important herb for female ailments, protects against contagious diseases and plagues, insecticide, hair tonic, as a bitter it stimulates the digestive process, fevers, infections.

Uses - Treatment of all worms, failing appetite, gastritis, gastric ulcers,, acidity, enteritis, constipation, jaundice, TB, tumor, pneumonia, pleurisy, all female ailments and bladder problems.

Externally - Prevention of falling hair, insecticide especially lice, sores, mange, inflammation of the ear, conjunctivitis.

Human Dose - 1 to 4mls of tincture 3 time a day.

Yarrow

Actions - Diaphoretic, astringent, diuretic, antiseptic, hypotensive.

It is a famed wound herb for staunching excess bleeding and derives it name from the Greek Warrior Achilles who healed his wounds and those of his soldiers with yarrow blossoms.

The herb is one of the best diaphoretics known to herbalists opening the skin pores and inducing lavish perspiration, sheep seek out the herb on dry ground as a food tonic, fevers, as a urinary antiseptic it can be used for cystitis, specific in thrombotic conditions associated with high blood pressure.

Uses - Treatment of all fevers, pneumonia, pleurisy, inflamed throat, hemorrhage's, uterine hemorrhages, dysentery, hysteria, epilepsy, rheumatism, colic.

Externally - Wounds, skin eruptions, abscess, earache.

Human Dose - 2 to 4mls of tincture 3 times a day.

Yellow Dock

Actions - Alterative, Cholagogue, purgative, mild astringent.

A powerful blood purifier and astringent. It is used in treating all diseases of the blood and skin. Very high in iron, making it useful for treating anemia. It nourishes and detoxifies the liver and cleanses and enriches the blood.

Used extensively for skin complaints such as psoriasis, a mild acting remedy for the relief of constipation has an action on the gallbladder.

Uses - Constipation, skin problems, gallbladder problems, jaundice.

Human Dose - 1 to 4mls of tincture 3 times a day.

Horse - 1 tablespoon of powder twice daily, less if purgative action is to much.

Yucca

Actions - Alterative, anti-inflammatory, anti-rheumatic ,laxative.

This herb is gaining attention for its treatment in dogs for arthritis, hip displasia and other degenerative hip and bone diseases. It seems to have a natural anti-inflammatory effect on the body. The saponins in

Yucca mimic the structure and effects of cortisone. Also aids in digestion and is a blood cleanser. Is now being used for gout.

Cautions - Use only the dried root. Long time use may impair the assimilation of the fat soluble vitamins.

Index of Herbal Actions

Adaptogen - Helps the body overcome its problems and work to the best of its ability. Good for overcoming the problems of chronic diseases, adapts the body to get the best it can out of itself. A good convalescent herb.

Herbs - Astragalus, Ginseng, Withania.

Alterative - Herbs that gradually restore proper function to the body, they increase health and vitality. They treat the toxicity of the blood and try to clean and purify the system. They were once known as the blood cleansers.

Herbs - Barberry, Black Cohosh, Blue Flag, Burdock, Cleavers, Chaparral, Devils Claw, Dong Quai, Echinacea, Figwort, Fumitory, Garlic, Nettles, Pau D'Arco ,Red Clover, Sarsaparilla, Sweet Violets, Yellow Dock, Wood Betony, Yucca.

Analgesic - Herbs that reduce pain.
Herbs - Chamomile, Devils Claw, Dong Quai, Hops, Meadowsweet, Pau D'Arco, Passion Flower,

Peppermint, Skullcap, St Johns Wort, Valerian, Withania, Willow Bark, Wood Betony.

Anti-biotic - Barberry, Chaparral, Echinacea, Elecampane, Garlic, Myrrh, Pau D' Arco, Plantain, Reshi, Tea Tree Oil.

Anti-catarrhal - Helps the body to remove excess catarrhal build ups.
Herbs - Cayenne, Coltsfoot, Cranesbill, Echinacea, Elder, Eyebright, Garlic, Golden Rod, Hyssop, Marshmallow, Mullein, Myrrh, Peppermint, Sage, Thyme, Yarrow.

Anti-emetic - Can reduce a feeling of nausea and can help to relieve or prevent vomiting.
Herbs - Barberry, Cayenne, Fennel, Meadowsweet, Peppermint.

Anti-fungal - Calendula, Cats Claw, Pau D' Arco, Myrrh, Sweet Violets.

Anti-inflammatory - Helps the body to combat inflammations. Herbs mentioned under demulcents, emollients and vulneraries will often act in this way especially when they are applied externally.
Herbs - Arnica, Blue Flag, Boswella, Cats Claw, Chaparral ,Chickweed, Cleavers, Cranesbill, Chamomile, Devils Claw, Eyebright, Feverfew, Ginger, Golden Rod, Guaiacum, Ladys Mantle,

Licorice, Marshmallow, Meadowsweet, Marigold, Pau D' Arco, St Johns Wort, Reshi, Sweet Violets, Willow Bark, Witch Hazel, Wormwood, Wild Yam, Yucca.

Anti-lithic - Prevent the formation of stones or gravel in the urinary system and help the body to remove them.
Herbs - Bearberry, Corn Silk, Chaparral Gravel Root.

Anti-microbial - Helps the body destroy or resist pathogenic micro-organisms.
Herbs - Aniseed, Cayenne, Cats Claw, Echinacea, Garlic, Gentian, Juniper, Marigold, Myrrh, Nasturtium, Peppermint, Plantain, Rosemary, Rue, Sage, Thyme, wormwood.

Anti-oxidant - Cats Claw, Chaparral, Garlic, Ginkgo Biloba, Hawthorn, Pau D'Arco

Anti-Rheumatic - Angelica, Burdock, Black Cohosh, Chaparral, Cats Claw, Celery Seed, Dandelion, Garlic, Guaiacum, Nettles, Willow Bark, Yellow Dock, Willow Bark, Wild Yam, Yucca.

Anti-Tumor - Burdock, Cleavers, Reshi, Poke Root, Shitake, Sweet Violets, Withania.

Antispasmodic - Prevents or eases spasms and

cramps.

Herbs - Aniseed, Angelica, Black Cohosh, Cat Mint, Chamomile, Dong Quai, Fennel, Grindelia, Horehound, Hyssop, Lemon Balm, Lime Blossom, Mistletoe, Motherwort, Passion Flower, Rosemary, Rue, Sage, Skullcap, St johns Wort, Thyme, Valerian, Vervain, Wild Yam, Wood Betony.

Anti-viral - Astragalus, Cats claw, Echinacea, Garlic, Lemon Balm, Myrrh?, Shitake, St Johns Wort, Pau D'Arco.

Anthelmintic - Destroys or expels worms from the digestive system.

Herbs - Centaury, Elecampane, Garlic, Nasturtium, Rue, Tansy, Thyme, Wormwood.

Aperient - Mild laxative.

Herbs - Burdock, Dandelion, Figwort, Rose Hips.

Astringent - Contracts tissue which in turn reduces discharges, these herbs contain tannins.

Herbs - Agrimony, Bear Berry, Cat Mint, Cranesbill, Chaparral, Chickweed, Comfrey, Eyebright, Golden Rod, Hops, Horsetail, Ladys Mantle, Marigold, Marshmallow, Meadowsweet, mullein, myrrh, Nettles, Plantain, Raspberry, Sage, Rosemary, Slippery Elm, Shepherds Purse, St Johns Wort, Slippery Elm, Thyme, Witch Hazel, Willow Bark, Wood Betony, Yarrow.

Bitter - Herbs that taste bitter act as stimulating tonics for the digestive system.
Herbs -Barberry, Burdock, Centaury, Feverfew, Gentian, Hops, Horehound, Rue, Tansy, Willow Bark, Wood Betony, Wormwood.

Carminative - Stimulates peristalsis of the digestive system and relaxes the stomach and helps remove gas and wind from the system. These herbs are usually rich in volatile oils.
Herbs - Aniseed, Angelica, Cat Mint, Cayenne, Chamomile, Fennel, Garlic, Ginger, Golden Rod, Hyssop, Horseradish, Juniper, Lemon Balm, Parsley, Peppermint, Penny Royal, Sage, Rosemary, Tansy, Thyme, Valerian, Wormwood.

Cardioactive - Has an effect on the heart.
Herbs - Broom, Figwort, Grindelia, Hawthorn, Lime Blossoms, Mistletoe, Motherwort.

Circulatory Tonic
Herbs - Ginger, Ginko Biloba, Hawthorn, Horse Chestnut, Wood Betony.

Cholagogue - Stimulates the release of bile from the gallbladder which can relieve gallbladder problems, bile is also the body's natural laxative so cholagogues have a laxative effect as well.
Herbs - Agrimony, Barberry, Blue Flag, Calendula,

Centaury, Dandelion, Fumitory, Gentian, Marigold, Milk Thistle, Yellow Dock.

Demulcent - Soothes and protects irritated or inflamed internal tissues.
Herbs - Bear Berry, Corn Silk, Coltsfoot, Comfrey, Fenugreek, Licorice, Marshmallow, Milk Thistle, Mullein, Oats, Plantain, Slippery Elm.

Diaphoretic - Aids the skin in the elimination of toxins and produces sweat thus reducing the temperature of fevers.
Herbs - Angelica, Black Cohosh, Cat Mint, Cayenne, Chamomile, Elder, Elecampane, Fennel, Garlic, Ginger, Golden Rod, Guaiacum, Hyssop, Lemon Balm, Lime Blossom, Peppermint, Sarsaparilla, Thyme, Vervain, Yarrow.

Diuretic - Increases the secretion and elimination of urine. Always give some demulcent herbs with diuretics so as to buffer the effect on the kidneys.
Herbs - Agrimony Angelica, Bear Berry, Blue Flag, Burdock, Buchu, Broom, Coltsfoot, Chaparral, Corn Silk, Dandelion Leaves, Elder, Figwort, Fumitory, Golden Rod, Guaiacum, Gravel Root, Grindelia, Hawthorn, Horseradish, Horsetail, Juniper, Lime Blossom, Nettles, Pau D' Arco, Penny Royal, Plantain, Parsley, Shepherds Purse, Sarsaparilla, Wood Betony, Yarrow.

Emmenagogue - Stimulates and normalizes the

menstrual flow, the cycle and are tonics for the female reproductive system.

Herbs - Black Cohosh, Chamomile, Chaste Tree, Dong Quai, Fenugreek, Gentian, Ginger, Juniper, Ladys Mantle, Lemon Balm, Marigold, Motherwort, Parsley, Penny Royal, Peppermint, Parsley, Raspberry, Sage, Rosemary, Rue, Shepherds Purse, St Johns Wort, Tansy, Thyme, Valerian, Vervain, Wormwood, Yarrow.

Emollient - Soothing to the skin. Acts externally the way demulcents do internally.

Herbs - Chickweed, Coltsfoot, Comfrey, Fenugreek, Licorice, Marshmallow, Mullein, Plantain, Slippery Elm.

Expectorant - Supports the body in the removal of excess mucous from the respiratory system and helps in the control of coughs.

Herbs -Angelica, Aniseed, Coltsfoot, Comfrey, Elder, Elecampane, Fennel, Fenugreek, Garlic, Grindelia, Hyssop, Horehound, Licorice, Marshmallow, Mullein, Myrrh, Nasturtium, Plantain, Red Clover, Sweet Violets, Thyme, Vervain.

Febrifuge - Helps the body to bring down fevers.

Herbs - Cayenne, Elder Flowers, Hyssop, Marigold, Penny Royal, Peppermint, Plantain, Raspberry, Sage, Thyme, Vervain, Willow Bark.

Galactagogue - Helps increase the flow of milk in females.
Herbs - Aniseed, Chaste Tree, Fennel, Fenugreek, Milk Thistle, Raspberry, Vervain.

Hypotensive - Lowers blood pressure.
Herbs - Astragalus, Barberry, Grindelia, Goldenrod, Hawthorn, Lemon Balm, Mistletoe, Passion Flower, Yarrow

Hypertensive - Raises Blood Pressure.
Herbs - Broom, Ginseng, Hawthorn (more of a balancer as it does both))

Hepatic - Tones and strengthens the liver, may increase the flow of bile.
Herbs - Agrimony, Blue Flag, Dandelion, Devils Claw, Fennel, Fumitory, Gentian, Horseradish, Hyssop, Motherwort, Milk Thistle, Vervain, Wormwood, Yarrow.

Hormone Balancers - Black Cohosh, Chaste Tree, Dong Quai, Withania

Immune Boosters - Astragalus, Echinacea, Myrrh, Reshi, Shitake.

Laxative - Promotes the evacuation of the bowels.
Herbs - Barberry, Burdock, Dandelion., Fumitory,

Horseradish, Licorice, Yucca.

Nervine - Has a beneficial effect on the nervous system, acts like a tonic to this system.
Herbs - Black Cohosh, Chamomile, Hops, Lime Blossoms, Mistletoe, Motherwort, Oats, Peppermint, Rosemary, Skullcap, St Johns Wort, Tansy, Thyme, Valerian, Vervain, Wormwood.

Parasiticide - Kills parasites and insects.
Herbs - Aniseed, Neem, Garlic, Rosemary, Elder (externally)

Pectoral - Has a general strengthening and healing effect on the respiratory system.
Herbs - Aniseed, Coltsfoot, Comfrey, Elder, Garlic, Hyssop, Licorice, Marshmallow, Mullein, Vervain, Horehound.

Rubefacient - Causes a gentle local irritation to the skin which stimulates the capillaries to open increasing the blood flow.
Herbs - Cayenne, Garlic, Ginger, Horseradish, Nettles, Peppermint Oil, Rosemary Oil, Rue.

Sialagogue - Stimulates the secretion of saliva.
Herbs - Blue flag, Cayenne, Gentian, Ginger.

Sedative - Calms the nervous system and reduces stress and nervousness throughout the body.

Herbs - Black Cohosh, Cat Mint, Chamomile, Hops, Hyssop, Motherwort, Passion Flower, Skullcap, St Johns Wort, Valerian , Vervain Wood Betony.

Stimulants - Quicken and enliven the physiological function of the body.
Herbs - Cayenne, Dandelion, Fennel, Garlic, Gentian, Ginger, Horseradish, Juniper, Penny Royal, Peppermint, Rosemary, Rue, Sage, Tansy, Horehound, Wormwood, Yarrow.

Tonics - Strengthen and enliven specific organs or the whole body.
Herbs - Agrimony, Aniseed, Black Cohosh, Burdock, Cayenne, Chamomile, Cleavers, Coltsfoot, Comfrey, Cranesbill, Corn Silk, Dandelion, Echinacea, Eyebright, Fumitory, Fenugreek, Gentian, Grindelia, Hawthorn, Lemon Balm, Liquorice, Mistletoe, Motherwort, Myrrh, Nettle, Oats, Parsley, Raspberry, Rue, Sarsaparilla, Skullcap, Tansy, Thyme, Vervain, Wormwood, Yarrow.

Urinary Antiseptics - Helps eliminate bacteria as it passes through the urinary tract.
Herbs - Bear Berry, Buchu, Cranberry,

Vermifuge - An agent that causes the expulsion of intestinal worms, see anthelmintics.

Vulnerary - Applied externally and aid the body in

the healing of wounds and cuts.

Herbs - Arnica, Burdock, Calendula, Chickweed, Comfrey, Cranesbill, Elder, Fenugreek, Garlic, Horsetail, Hyssop, Marigolds, Marshmallow, Mullein, Myrrh, Plantain, Shepherds Purse, Slippery Elm, St Johns Wort, Thyme, Witch Hazel, Yarrow.

Homeopathic Supplement

Homeopathy has been around now for hundreds of years and unlike most other forms of medicine its rules have not changed and will not for they are based on a essential truth. The main rule is Like cures Like or if we break down the word Homeopathy homo means the same and pathy means disease. As Homoeopathy is a very hard science to learn and as it kind of sits or balances on the border of hard science and metaphysics I will not try to explain to you what it is here as it would probably take a whole book to do this but I will say this, in the UK and a lot of countries in Europe it is on and paid for by the National Health System and anything that can get a politician to open their purse must work.

It is said that Homeopathy sits on a three legged stool. What this means is that if a remedy has at least three symptoms in the same strength as the symptoms you are trying to match then that remedy is a potential cure for your condition or if not cure it will offer the condition relief. The more symptoms you can match to the remedy the better the remedy will work for the rule is likes cure likes not vaguely similar cures. Listed below are some common Homoeopathic Remedies and some of the symptoms they cover. The idea is to find one remedy that covers most of your symptoms. To make the remedies as closer a match as we can we ask lots of questions like the ones below and after we gather all the answers we have what is called a good Symptom Picture which we then try to match as accurately as we can to a Remedy. Most Homeopathic Materia Medicas are set out to answer the questions listed below with the mind symptoms being the most important. Questions on time, position and temperature are good for making a choice between to very close remedies. The best Materia Medica for the lay person is Boerickes and you should be able to view this on a few Homeopathic websites.

Symptom Guide Questions

1/. Was there a sudden onset of the condition, at what time?

2/. What time of the day does the patient feel either better or worse.

3/. What is the effect of motion? jarring? walking? running?

4/. What is the effect of drinking fluids? warm and or cold drinks?

5/. Is the patient thirsty or not at all? sips or gulps?

6/. Is the onset from exertion? overeating? weather changes? emotions?

7/. Mental emotional state of patient?

8/. Better warm room? warm air?

9/. Better cool room? cool open air?

10/. Are the respirations upper chest movements or in the abdomen?

11/. Respirations - dry or wet?

12/. Expectoration - watery or stringy mucous, easy or difficult.

13/. Is there coughing

14/. Position - better or worse from sitting? standing? lying? lying on which side?

15/. Along with the condition is there fever? gas? belching? wind?

Modality - The questions above are covering what the Homoeopaths call modalities which basically mean are covering a condition that makes the patient better or worse. I will list the main Modalities below. The Modalities help us to distinguish which remedy is right for the case especially when we have a group that look as though they may all work which is what I am giving you und the disease heading. Using modalities forces you to think what really is going on, is this the nature of the beast or the nature of the disease.

Time - Better or Worse morning, night, weekly, monthly, seasonally etc.

Motion - Better or Worse first movement, rest, exertion, walking, stretching, rising up etc

Temperature - Better or Worse heat, cold, cold air blowing, sudden change etc.

Body Activity - Better or Worse eating, drinking,

urinating, defecating, sleep, coughing etc

Weather - - Better or Worse, damp, sunny, foggy, storms, sudden changes etc.

Senses - Better or Worse - touch, pressure, noise, light, odors etc.

Position - Better or Worse lying, standing, sitting, stretched out, doubled up, right side etc.

Mind - Excitement, anger, fear, stress, better busy, nervous all the time etc.

Now read through all the remedies in the Marteria Medica (Homoeopathic Remedy Reference) and you will notice that most of them have Mind or mental symptoms kind of describing the personalities or moods a good example is Nux Vomica, I think we all know a nasty type of individual that this remedy would be suited to and meaning as though the individual is suited to this remedy then the remedy would have a curative action on them but don't expect it to change the nature of the beast. One of the main rules of Homeopathy is the closer the match of the remedy the higher the Potency you use but if you are not used to Homoeopathy just use the 30C potency and remember what I said about the 3 legged stool. Potency is a measure of strength and depth of action.

Remember as mentioned before Homoeopathy sits on a three legged stool. What this means is that if a remedy has at least three symptoms in the same strength as your symptoms then that remedy is a potential cure.

Note - The best prescribing guide for the layman is **Boerickes Materia Medica With Repertory.**
Another good guide is **The Complete Book Of Homeopathy by Dr Michael Weiner.**
I always buy my books on Homeopathy from India as they are quarter the price and there is always a wide selection. Put B. Jain Publishers into the google search engine go to their web site and check out these books and I am sure you will be pleased with what you find.

Disease Nosodes

Nosodes are remedies made from disease material mainly from the tissues, discharges, exudates, excretions, suppurations or secretions of a infected being. Simply stated a Nosode is a homeopathic remedy prepared from a pathological specimen. Rabies Nosode, for example starts with the saliva of a rabid dog and is then potentized.

Nosodes have many uses and are widely used in homeopathic practice to help limit cases of infectious diseases and to help during the recovery phase of a disease especially the ones that linger and drag on. There are Nosodes for most infectious diseases of animals and humans the use of Nosodes in this way is referred to as isopathy rather than Homoeopathy. They are often used in farm situations, to limit the spread and the effects of infectious diseases. This has especially been used as a vital component of mastitis control on many farms, both organic and conventional. One documented event about Nosodes dates back to Napoleon marching his Legions through Europe and spreading Typhoid in their wake, the towns that had the best cure rates were the ones where the local Homoeopaths used a Nosode of the disease.

Nosodes can be used in the prevention of infectious diseases in the manner of vaccination but they work by a completely different mechanism then from the raising of antibodies that vaccines work by. As yet it is not actually known how they work but they have survived hundreds of years ridicule by producing results and will carry on doing so.

The best known study into Nosodes was done by Dr. Christopher Day of England involving 'kennel cough' in a boarding kennel. At the time he was called in, there were 40 dogs in the kennel with 35 that had kennel cough. About half had been vaccinated for this malady. He gave a Nosode to all the animals that were there and all the dogs that came in through the rest of the summer, which was another 214 dogs. He successfully reduced the incidence of kennel cough from over 90% to less than 2%.

Nosodes used for the prevention of diseases are usually given in the 30C potency. A good dosing regime is one dose given night and morning for 3 days followed by one per month for the next 6 months. This generally provides a good level of protection after the first week. A good example of how this can be used is a puppy given the Nosode of Parvovirus at 3 to 4 weeks of age instead of having to wait for 9 weeks for the vaccination, this way the puppy is protected before given the vaccination.

Nosodes can have homeopathic therapeutic properties in their own right. Such Nosodes are found in the Homoeopathic Materia Medica and have undergone a proper 'proving'. Examples are Bacillinum, Carcinosinum, Medorrhinum, Psorinum, Tuberculinum.

Dose - Dr. Surjit S. Makker recommends 20ml of remedy mixed with 8 liters of water for 100 birds. This medicated water should be shaken well and put in drinkers accordingly. For individual birds give them 2-3 pellets by mouth and keep them calm.

How To Make A Nosode In A Hurry

This is not the right way of making a Homoeopathic preparation but it is an effective way when you have an emergency situation and have to react fast.

1/. Get a sample of the pathogen you need from the patient, for example, Pus from a wound or popular eruption,, sputum coughed up from the lungs or any other disease product, it can even be the scrapings from a stubborn ringworm infection that won't go away. Sometimes the more sources of the same disease combined e.g. sputum and pus from an eruption the better the result.

2/. Find a clean 600ml jar and sterilize it by putting it in the oven at a high temperature for a while as you would for sterilizing preserving jars. After the jar is sterilized place your disease products in and fill with sterilized water or distilled water which is cheap and easy to buy from an auto shop as they use it in batteries. Shake the jar for a while until you are sure the mixture is dissolved.

3/. Empty the jar, there will always be a residue from whatever sticks to the sides and you will see the drops gather again at the bottom of the jar after it is upright.

4/. Fill the jar again with distilled water, this time at about 500mls. This will become our first potency. Get a book and put it on a table and sit down and get comfortable. We are going to gently bang the jar against the book for 100 percussions. Homoeopathic remedies are energy medicines; we are imprinting our disease products onto the universal medium, water.

5/. Repeat steps 3 and 4 again for 27 times bringing our remedy close to a normal 30C homoeopathic potency, now you can see why I told you to sit down and get comfortable.

6/. On the 29 time use half and half water and vodka. We still have one more to go after this but we are going to save most of this as a stock to make more if needed. This is very important especially in cases of epidemics where you can give your friends and others some of this and they only have to percuss a part of this 100 times to get the needed nosode for medicating others and themselves.

7/. Make the last potency again in half water and half vodka. This is our last potency to make for we are as close as we can get to the 30C potency by doing it this way. The dose will be 10 drops under the tongue 3 times a day as a preventative or 5 drops every 30 minutes at the beginning of an acute infection. Take the normal precautions used with Homoeopathic Potencies i.e. no coffee or anything strong half an hour before or after the remedy.

Materia Medica

Note - All Homeopathic Remedies are given in Potency and not in material Form.

Aconite

Characteristics - Aconite is best used in the first stages of a illness, especially when fear and anxiety are present. Symptoms appear suddenly, without warning and they may be caused by exposure to cold winds or draughts or by a severe fright. Symptoms are a marked restlessness, animal displays extreme anxiety or fear, high fever with a burning skin, extreme sweating and a burning thirst, a hoarse dry painful cough, bright light noises stress and cold worsen the symptoms, rest and quiet relieves the symptoms. The pains of Aconite are unbearable, sharp, shooting, burning pains, tingling and numbness. A remedy for fevers and inflammatory states, use at the first sign of all fevers, shivering with cold sweats, difficult breathing, animal shows desire for large quantities of water, symptoms worse at midnight, symptoms improve in the open air.

Mind - Great fear, anxiety, restlessness, extreme sensitivity to pain, worry, foreboding.

Better - In open air, warmth, rest.

Worse - In the evening and night, particularly before midnight, lying on affected side.

Allium Cepa

Characteristics - Increased secretions from the eyes and nose, like those of the common cold. Frequent sneezing with watery discharge which burns the nose and upper lip, but the eye discharge is bland and doesn't burn (the opposite of Euphrasia). Tickling in the throat with incessant cough (feels as if larynx is split) holds throat when coughing. Being in cool open air relieves the symptoms, eyelids are swollen and red, abdominal tympany with wind, this remedy is indicated in the early stages of most catarrhal conditions, mild forms of cat flu can be cut short if given early.

Better - Cold room (except cough), open air.

Worse - Evening, warm room, odors.

Antimonium Tartaricum - Ant Tart

Characteristics - Is characterized by a loose rattling unproductive cough such as is often herd in cats. Respiration can be very difficult with much gasping. There is usually thirst for little and often. Symptoms are worse in the evening, lying down and in cold damp weather or a warm room. Confined largely to respiratory diseases, abundant bronchial secretions, great rattling of mucous with little expectoration, drowsiness, debility and sweat.

Mind - Drowsy and despondent, fear of being alone, child will not be touched without whining.

Better - Sitting erect, from burping and expectoration.

Worse - Evenings, lying down, damp cold weather.

Apis

Characteristics - Apis is used for various types of swelling and inflammation such as that from animal bites and bites and stings from insects, it is also used for measles, mumps, sore throats, sore red eyes and fever. Apis is a quick acting remedy for inflammations especially those ones with edema and lots of swelling which is its main use. Acute nephritis with scanty and burning urine there may be some blood in the urine. . Symptoms are swelling with edema which makes the effected parts look shiny, red and puffy, the swollen parts feel soggy and waterlogged, a fever that develops rapidly but without thirst, extreme restlessness and fidgeting, an irritable nature and perhaps jealous, cool air and cold compresses relieve the symptoms. Pains are burning and stinging, arthritis with swelling, animals seek cold surface to lie on, swollen eyelids, may be swollen ears, may be blood in the urine, in the horse and cow there may be edema in the lower limbs while in dogs abdominal dropsy is seen. Symptoms get worse from heat and improve in the open air and from cold bathing.

Mind - Apathy, indifference, awkward.

Better - By cold, (room, air or application)

Worse - From warmth, pressure, late in the afternoon, from sleeping.

Arnica

Characteristics - Bruises and similar injuries where the skin is unbroken and there is mental or emotional shock. Symptoms are any type of bruising or similar injury caused by crushing, squeezing or wrenching, muscles strains which feel sore and bruised, shock after accidents, there is a fear of being touched because of the pain, good for the soreness after birth and medical operations.

Arnica can be used in potency and also as a cream. The cream must not be used on broken skin or wounds. Animal shrinks away when you try to touch it, symptoms improve when lying down.

Mind - Fears touch or approach, whole body oversensitive.

Better - Lying down or with head low.

Worse - Least touch, motion, damp and cold.

Arsenic Album

Characteristics - Burning pains relieved by heat, anxious, restless, weak and chilly with an air of fear and hopelessness. Anxiety or restlessness are often present where this remedy is indicated. Discharge from eyes and nose are watery and acrid causing ulceration in those regions. The mouth is usually dry and the patient is usually thirsty. Dramatic vomiting and diarrhea often simultaneously indicate its use if the modalities agree. The patient may have wheezing respiration and allergic asthmatic conditions can respond well. The skin can be dry, scaly and scruffy. Symptoms are worse for cold and wet better for warmth. Tries to find relief in motion but immediately feels weak with movement. Restless, feels cold, complains of general weakness, discharges burn the skin.

Mind - Fear with despair and restlessness.

Better - Warmth, open air, relieved by sweat, hot drinks, lying down (but restless).

Worse - Cold air, after midnight eg 1 to 3am. Wet damp weather and near sea shore.

Belladonna

Characteristics - This is one of the great fever remedies, conditions requiring its use usually being of violent and sudden onset. Heat, redness, pain and swelling characterize its symptoms. It is one of the main remedies used in convulsions. Pupils are usually dilated which is a keynote for this remedy. Acute ear inflammation where there is heat, pain and swelling respond well. The mouth is usually dry and there is great thirst. With Belladonna always think BIRDS. B for burning, I for irritability, R for redness,

D for delirium and S for spasms.

Mind - Hallucinations, delirium, rages, bites, strikes, desire to escape.

Better - For quiet, dark, rest with slight warmth.

Worse - For noise, touch or jarring motion.

Bellis Perennis

Characteristics - Trauma to abdomen and pelvic organs especially after surgery and child birth if arnica does not give relief. Injuries to the nerves with intense soreness, back ache from hard physical work such as gardening, pain is bruised sore and aching, better cold presses, worse touch, after getting wet.

The animal is unwilling to move and when made to do so evidences pain, muscular stiffness is prominent.

Worse - Left side and cold wind.

Bryonia

Characteristics - This remedy shows both diarrhea and constipation symptoms, the latter usually in chronic conditions. The mouth is often dry and there is great thirst. The tongue is often coated yellow. It is of great help in many cases of rheumatism or arthritis where the symptoms agree. There is often respiratory signs with a hoarse hacking cough. All symptoms are worse for movement and better for rest.

Mind - Irritable, delirium.

Better - Lying on the painful side, pressure, rest and cold things.

Worse - Warmth, motion, morning, eating and touch.

Calendula

Characteristics - The part used is the Flowers and it is used for wounds and skin irritations, it is healing, soothing, anti-inflammatory, astringent, anti-fungal and anti-microbial.

Use as a lotion for cuts, grazes, infected sores, fungal infections, any skin inflammations, regulates the oil production of the skin so is good for acne, to stop bleeding, for bruises and sprains, skin ulcers and minor burns and scolds.

Note - The tincture of this is used as a lotion diluted at 1 to 10.

Cantharis

Characteristics - Important first aid remedy for minor burns and for other pains that feel burning and fiery, also has a healing effect on the bladder, urethra and other parts of the urinary tract where burning pain is the key symptom, burns and scalds especially where blistering and inflammation occur, sunburn, insect bites that feel hot and burn, cystitis. Pains are violent burning, cutting, stabbing or smarting, rawness, use when the animal appears distressed when passing urine, or tries to pass and cannot. Better from warmth rest and rubbing.

Mind - Furious delirium, acute mania generally of a

sexual type, crying, barking.

Better - From rubbing

Worse - From touch or approach, from urinating, from drinking cold water.

Carbo Vegetabilis

Characteristics - Patient exhibits mental and physical sluggishness and symptoms come on slowly, generalized weakness of all functions especially digestion, overweight, torpid, lazy, complaints of coldness, pains usually described as burning, pressing pains, wishes to be fanned, digestive problems such as belching often accompany any illness.

Mind - Aversion to darkness, sudden loss of memory.

Better - Being fanned, passing gas, rest.

Worse - Morning and evening, exertion, cold, tight clothes at abdomen.

Causticum

Characteristics - Burns and burning pains such as cystitis also used for dry coughs, burns to the skin especially with marked inflammation and blistering, coughs, laryngitis and hoarseness from straining and over using voice, cystitis especially with involuntary passing of urine when coughing, chronic cystitis, exposure to cold dry air may make symptoms worse.

Mind - Least thing makes it cry, sad, hopeless. Ailments from long lasting grief.

Better - In damp wet weather, warmth.
Worse - Cold winds.

Euphrasia

Characteristics - Affects the mucous membranes of the eyes, nose and chest producing copious watery secretions,eye secretions cause smarting of the skin while the nose discharge is bland. Used for conjunctivitis, eye strain generally but especially from computers, eyes that feel sore and inflamed and look red, hay fever symptoms including a tickly throat, sneezing, a runny nose, and itchy red watering eyes. Sunlight wind and warmth worsen the symptoms. Use for Dogs who have had their head out of the window for too long, symptoms better in dim light or darkness, in all species a tendency to diarrhea occurs.

Better - In the dark

Worse - From light, indoors, in the evening.

Hypericum

Characteristics - Used for bruises and other injuries especially to nerve rich areas like the fingers, lips, ears, eyes ,tail bone, good for the pain of puncture wounds of any cause eg animal or insect. Helps with the pains after operations especially amputations. Pains are violent shooting pains along a nerve path, burning, tingling and numbness. Worse from shock and touch and better from rubbing, horse fly bites, symptoms worse cold better warmth.

Mind - Anxiety, melancholy, effects of shock.

Better - Bending head backward.

Worse - Cold, dampness and touch.

Ipecac

Characteristics - Indicated for complaints of persistent nausea not relieved by vomiting, ailments caused by eating rich or indigestible type of foods such as ice-cream, sweets etc., useful to stop bleeding if blood is bright red.

Mind - Easily irritated, child cries or screams continuously, wanting something but not sure what they desire, holds everything in contempt.

Worse - Warm, moist weather, lying down.

Kali Bichromicum

Characteristics - Has a affinity for the mucous membranes of the body, tough stringy viscid secretions sometimes forming thick yellow green mucous, sinus infections, suited for fleshy fat light complexioned people, general weakness.

Better - Heat

Worse - Cold, beer, morning, undressing.

Kali Carbonicum

Characteristics - Has a affinity for the mucous membranes digestive and respiratory, very tired, anemic, flabby tissues which may be swollen, sweat, backache, weakness, many conditions have a aggravation at 2am to 4am, often stays immobile when ill.

Mind - Very irritable, hypersensitive to pain, despondent.

Better - During the day, sitting down, bending forward, warmth.

Worse - Cold weather, between 2am and 4am.

Lachesis

Characteristics - Many symptoms tend to be left sided, cannot bear tight clothing, symptoms worse on awakening, symptoms relieved with onset of the menstrual flow. Short dry cough, feels relief after coughing up watery phlegm, feeling of constriction in throat and chest, better bending forward.

Mind - Overly talkative, impatient, sad, jealous, no desire to mix with world.

Better - Release of pressure, eating fruit, cold, discharges.

Worse - Pressure, touch, after sleep, heat, hot weather.

Ledum

Characteristics - Has a action on the capillaries and is useful for cleaning up bruises especially around the eyes, mainly used for puncture wounds made by sharp points such as nails and wood splinters and insect bites and stings especially ones that don't heal properly and look blue and puffy. Wounds that feel cold to the touch, septic conditions, sprains, pains are throbbing, tearing ,prickling, they shoot upwards, stiff and sore. Better cold, cold bathing. This remedy was used in the past along with hypericum to ward off tetanus especially in deep wounds

Better - From cold.

Worse - At night and from heat.

Lycopodium

Characteristics - Exerts most of its effects on the digestive organs, liver, kidneys and respiratory systems. The patient dislikes being left alone and appears apprehensive. The nose is often blocked and there may be blisters on the tongue. Eating a little food always satisfies the appetite but appetite is very marked. The belly is usually bloated. The stool appears hard and small and is expelled only with difficulty accompanied by ineffectual straining. Urination is also a slow process and the urine has a red sediment. Symptoms are worse for heat generally and better for cold.

Mind - Melancholy, afraid to be alone, apprehensive.

Better - By motion, on getting cold.

Worse - From heat.

Natrum Sulphuricum

Characteristics - A good liver remedy, emotional

and mental difficulties arising after head injury, useful in problems associated with rainy weather and dampness, patient feels every change from dry to wet weather, may remove excess water and fluid retention from the body.

Mind - Lively music saddens, melancholy, inability to think, dislikes to speak or be spoken to.

Better - Dry weather and environments, pressure, change of position.

Worse - Damp weather, damp basements, lying on left side.

Nux Vom

Characteristics - The remedy for overindulgence, adapted especially to thin irritable energetic people who attend with great detail to tasks, quarrelsome, nervous, intelligent, hypochondriacal, oversensitive to noise music and light, craves stimulants.

Primarily used in the digestive sphere, its greatest reputation is in helping disturbances following overeating of unsuitable foods. Feces is usually hard but diarrhea can follow overeating. There is abdominal discomfort, flatulence, irritability and sensitivity to noise. Symptoms are generally worse for noise and better after rest or for damp weather.

Mind - Very irritable, sensitive to all impressions, malicious, disposed to reproach others.

Better - Wet weather, lying down, uninterrupted nap.

Worse - Overeating, mental over exertion, sensory stimulation ie sound, sight, touch etc.

Phosphorus

Characteristics - Irritated and inflamed mucous and serous membranes are the key feature of this remedy. Is a very sudden remedy with suddenness of symptoms. The patient is sensitive to loud and sudden noises (eg thunder fireworks etc). Degenerative processes and bone destruction respond well to Phosphorus. Food is suddenly vomited back up when it has been warmed in the stomach, gums can be ulcerated and bloody. Hepatitis, jaundice, pancreatic disease and nephritis come into its sphere. Urine may be bloody. A very painful cough is also a symptom. Wounds that perpetually bleed may also be helped. The patient is usually in poor body condition. Symptoms are worse for touch, exertion, in the evening and during thunder storm. Better for cold and sleep.

Mind - Low spirits, restless, fidgety.

Better - In the dark, lying on the right side, from the cold, sleep.

Worse - Touch, from exertion and in the evening.

Pulsatilla

Characteristics - Often indicated for those with mild, gentle, timid yielding dispositions who are easily moved to laughter and tears, The Pulsatilla person wants to be held and loved, moods changeable and fickle, the patient is chilly but desires strolling in cold air, symptoms are erratic and change frequently, pains are wandering, pains that grow gradually in intensity, fever without thirst despite dry mouth, bland yellow discharges.

Mind - Weeps easily, timid, fears to be alone - dark - ghosts, likes sympathy and fuss, highly emotional, easily discouraged, sensitive.

Better - Open air, cold applications, consolation relieves symptoms.

Worse - Evening before midnight, warmth, after eating fat rich food.

Rhus Tox

Characteristics - Is the most famous of the rheumatic remedies. The skin and muscular skeletal system are its main spheres. Small red papules in the skin and sometimes vesicles are typical lesions with much scratching. In all cases of damage to muscles think of Rhus and the symptoms of arthritis which are worse after rest particularly if this follows strenuous exertion. The symptoms improve with limbering up , The worst pains are seen as the animal arises from its bed.

Mind - Listless, sad, extreme restlessness, great apprehension at night.

Better - Warmth, walking, from stretching out limbs.

Worse - During sleep, cold wet rainy weather and at

night.

Ruta

Characteristics - Has effects on the joints, tendons, cartilages, and the periosteum which is a fine membrane that covers bones and gives it that shiny look, it is also used for eye strain where the vision goes dim.

Used for painful bruises affecting the bones, dislocations, strains to the tendons or joints, aching with restlessness, pains are gnawing, digging, burning, bruised, sore as if beaten, bones as if broken, pain deep in the bones, rheumatism.

Better - From lying and warmth.

Worse - From over exertion, touch, cold wet weather.

Silica

Characteristics - Fits the shy chilly patient who is reluctant to enter the room, chronic inflammatory conditions such as sinus, helps in the removal of foreign bodies such as splinters and seeds, ripens abscesses, ailments attended with pus formation. Use silica and be prepared to use it for a while sometimes up to 3 weeks.

Mind - Faint hearted, anxious, yielding.

Better - Warmth, wet or humid weather.

Worse - Morning, from lying down, cold.

Staphysagria

Characteristics - Suits sensitive people who suppress their feelings and suffer in silence or who boil over with indignation, remedy for cuts and wounds especially those that are from medical procedures and have the mentioned feelings. Nervous states of animals. The pains are stinging, stitching, smarting, squeezing, as if stabbed by a knife. Worse from touch, emotions and suppressed anger.

Better - Warmth, rest at night.

Worse - Touch on affected parts, loss of fluids.

Symphytum

Characteristics - Causes bone to grow and promotes fast healing should be given for all fractures. Used for injuries to the hard parts of the body while arnica is for the soft parts. Also used for eye injuries caused from blows.

Caution - do not use if a pin has been placed in the bone as the pin has to be removed latter.

Tarentula Cubensis

Characteristics - For abscesses, boils, carbuncles, swellings of any kind but especially on the back of the neck where the skin turns black, red/blue or purple with great pain. Deep septic conditions with hardening of the effected part, condition comes on fast, pains are burning, stinging, throbbing, pricking like a needle.

Worse - Night.

Urtica Urens

Characteristics - Can be used for burns and also for cystitis where the urine burns the skin and there is dificulty passing urine. Symptoms are stinging pains, swellings particularly blistery swellings, itching.

Worse - Cool moist air, touch.

The Safest Essential Oils For Animal Use

Extreme care must be taken using the Essential Oils on animals. The ones mentioned in these pages seem to be the safest if used in a low dose which is a quarter of what you would use on a human and even this would be too high if used on a mouse so really think about what you are doing and always use a little test dose to check for sensitivity.

Danger - Do not use on **birds** and **cats** as there metabolism cannot handle Essential oils and death will be the most likely result, this includes Eucalyptus and Tea Tree oil.

How Oils Work

Essential Oils work by entering the blood stream via the pores of the skin so the biggest action is on the area applied followed by a systemic action via the blood. The liver is the main blood filter and detoxifier of the body so the liver is responsible for breaking down any drug or blood borne foreigner so with the Essential Oils there is always the chance that if the dose is too high or the application is to frequent the liver may be damaged. Never forget that oils are highly concentrated products. A good example is a budgie, you clipped the wings and one is now bleeding so you put Tea Tree oil on it. Imagine the size of one drop of oil now imagine the size of a Budgies liver and it's fairly obvious what's going to happen.

Below are given the cautions for using oils on dogs, follow these cautions on all animals in general. Most information for these pages was sourced from Kristen Leigh Bells book Holistic Aromatherapy For Animals and Catharine Birds book A Healthy Horse The Natural Way.

Essential Oil Blends
Soothing Skin Essential Oil Blend
15ml base oil of hazel nut or sweet almond oil

2 drops Geranium

6 drops Rosewood

6 drops Lavender

1 drop Roman Chamomile

2 drops Carrot Seed

Combine all ingredients, shake and store in a dark glass bottle. Use 2 to 4 drops of this blend to spot treat small areas of skin.

Mange Treatment Blend
15ml base oil of hazel nut or sweet almond oil

5 drops Lavender

7 drops Niaouli

1 drop Helichrysum

2 drops Sweet Marjoram

After bathing the dog 2 to 4 drops of the blend should be applied to the affected areas twice a day for at least 2 weeks. Observe for a week and repeat if necessary. Try to prevent the dog from licking the area.

Tick Bite Forula

15ml base oil of hazel nut or sweet almond oil
5 drops Thyme Thujanol
3 drops Hyssop Decumbens
8 drops Lavender

For use on bites or immediately after the tick is removed to help prevent infection, reduce redness and inflammation and possibly prevent Lymes disease.

Fresh Breath Oil Blend

5ml base oil of hazel nut or sweet almond oil
6 drops Cardamom
4 drops Coriander Seed
6 drops Peppermint
1 to 3 drops inside of the dogs mouth.

Calm Dog Blend

15ml base oil of hazel nut or sweet almond oil
3 drops Valerian
2 drops Vetiver
4 drops Petitgrain
3 drops Sweet Marjoram
2 drops Sweet Orange

The calming effect ranges from taking the edge off to soothing the dog. Dose is 1 to 6 drops depending on the size of the dog.

Fear or Seperation Anxiety
15ml base oil of hazel nut or sweet almond oil
1 drop Neroli
2 drops Sweet Bazil
4 drops Bergamot
6 drops Petitgrain
1 drop Ylang Ylang
Dose is 1 to 6 drops depending on size of dog.

Flea Free Blend
15ml base oil of hazel nut or sweet almond oil
4 drops Clary Sage
1 drop Citronella
7 drops Peppermint
3 drops Lemon
Store in dark glass bottle. 2 to 4 drops to the neck, chest, legs and tail base of the dog.

Tick Free Blend
15ml base oil of hazel nut or sweet almond oil
2 drops Geranium
2 drops Rosewood
3 drops Lavender
2 drops Myrhh
2 drops Opoponax
1 drop Bay Leaf
Store in dark glass bottle. 2 to 4 drops to the neck, chest, legs and tail base of the dog.

Increasing The Appetite
15ml base oil of hazel nut or sweet almond oil

2 drops Sweet Orange
2 drops Lemon
2 drops Grapefruit
2 drops Lime
2 drops Bergamot
For old and sick dogs this is a gentle appetite stimulant. 2 to 6 drops of the final blend to the neck and chest of the dog gently rubbed in. Repeat as needed up to 6 times per day.

Immune Boosting Blend
15ml base oil of hazel nut or sweet almond oil
2 drops Bay Laurel
2 drops Ravensare
2 drops Palmarosa
2 drops Eucalyptus
2 drops Niaouli
2 drops Coriander Seed
2 drops Thyme Thujanol
2 to 4 drops daily via massage to neck and chest.

Colds and Congestion
15ml base oil of hazel nut or sweet almond oil
5 drops Eucalyptus
5 drops Myrhh
5 drops Ravensare
For relieving nasal congestion or cold symptoms in dogs. 1 to 6 drops rubbed into neck or chest.

Fatigue Blend
15ml base oil of hazel nut or sweet almond oil

7 drops Rosemary
6 drops Tangerine
3 drops Ylang Ylang
Balancing and revitalizing for dogs that are suffering from fatigue and malaise.
2 to 4 drops daily via massage to neck and chest.

Flatulence Blend
15ml base oil of hazel nut or sweet almond oil
3 drops Caraway
3 drops Cardamom
3 drops Cinnamon
3 drops Nutmeg
3 drops Tangerine
1 to 2 drops placed on your dog's food and then 1 or 2 drops given after eating. Many dogs enjoy the taste of this spicy blend and will lick it off your hand. The spice oils of this blend are commonly found in food flavorings so digestion is regarded as safe.

Joint Rub Blend
15ml base oil of hazel nut or sweet almond oil
3 drops Black Pepper
4 drops Peppermint
3 drops Speramint
4 drops Juniper Berry
Good for muscle soreness, arthritis, hip dysplasia and sprains. use 2 to 4 drops of the blend and try to rub in as close to the skin as possible. Do a patch test with this oil as it can be irritating. Patch tests can be done with drop of blend in the arm pit.

Motion Sickness Blend
15ml base oil of hazel nut or sweet almond oil
7 drops Ginger
8 drops Peppermint
Give 3 drops in the mouth

Labor Ease Blend
15ml base oil of hazel nut or sweet almond oil
6 drops Clary Sage
1 drop Neroli
5 drops Petitgrain
2 drops Lavender
1 drop Roman Chamomile
Calming and balancing blend, can be applied to the fur of the neck or chest or 1 to 4 drops can be rubbed in the belly.

Oils For Horses

The safest way to use Essential Oils on your horse are external massage and inhalation. When inhaled the Oil addresses the horses emotional states and stored memories as well as entering the body and having an effect with the most obvious here being Eucalyptus which acts as a bronchodilator (illegal for competition horses in some parts of the US). **Use blends in the same strengths as mentioned in dogs don't go over 2% oil in a blend. Only apply the** blends to the affected areas. You can copy some of the dog formulas or make your own using the list of oils.

Essential Oils For Animal Use

The Essential Oils below are fairly safe for Animal Use

Basil (Sweet) - Helpful for restoring mental balance and clarity. For animals that are suffering nervousness or anxiety, dogs with separation anxiety. Use sparingly (PMC30%). **Horses** - Helps to release most muscle spasms. Used before a event it minimizes the amount of uric acid in the blood and other toxic wastes from exercise. A warming winter oil feeding the muscle fibers and stimulating the blood flow. It is a expectorant removing mucous from a clogged respiratory system when rubbed into the chest and inhaled. Rubbed into the abdomen it may help to relieve the pain and symptoms of colic. May irritate the skin in high doses and don't use in pregnancy.

Bay Leaf - Good for a hair and fur tonic, ticks don't like it, good deodorizer.
Actions - Ant microbial.

Bay Laurel - Used in blends for boosting the immune system especially in dogs. Use only in small amounts in blends.

Bergamot - Combines toning, strengthening and balancing effects with soothing, relaxing and uplifting qualities. Useful for the treatment of fungal conditions such as dog ear infections due to yeast overgrowth. Use in small doses as it can cause photosensitization. **Horse** - Use full for treating any skin complaint especially folliculitis, flaking skin and wounds. Good for lice infections and bites, aids in the healing of any wounds and reduces scar formation. Has a stimulating effect on appetite. Be cautious when applying to the skin of a gray horse or to sensitive skin areas that will be exposed to the sun as this oil can cause photosensitization or pigment changes.

Black Pepper - Warming and circulatory stimulant qualities with low toxicity and irritation. Good for sore muscles, joint pains, arthritis and hip dysplasia. **Horse** - Gives tone to skeletal muscles and warms any winter chills. Dilates local blood vessels and improves local blood flow to the muscles warming the muscles from inside. Arthritic joints respond well to pepper and helps with pain management when used over a long period of time. Strengthens the nervous system. May antidote Homoeopathics.

Caraway Seed - Good for digestive problems, wind, poor appetite, indigestion and bad breath.

Cardamom - Digestive problems, bad breath. **Horse** - Good for treating digestive problems of a nervous origin. Encourages the flow of saliva and good for loss of appetite. It is warming when the body feels cold and useful for easing coughs and respiratory complaints. Highly antiviral and second only to

Eucalyptus in that respect. For stallions you can use it as an aphrodisiac. May irritate some sensitive skins.

Carrot Seed - Valuable oil in the use of skin care, dry flaky skin that is sensitive to allergens and prone to infections. **Horses** - Strengthens the mucous membranes so is good for respiratory conditions. Useful for regenerating the skin after wounds or skin diseases and it antiseptic action will deal with minor infections. Has a toning hormone like action that will encourage conception and assist the infertile mare.

Cedarwood Atlas - Gentle stimulating oil that increases circulation and stimulates the release toxins. Good for the skin and fleas don't like it. **Horse** - Sores that are slow to heal, saddle sores, folliculitis etc. and dry flaky skin, encourage the re-growth of coat and adds shine. Has a tonic effect on the kidneys. Dries out excess phlegm and runny noses and removes excess mucous from the respiratory system when inhaled.

Chamomile German - Powerful skin soothing ant inflammatory. Burns, allergic reaction and all types of skin irritations can be quickly calmed with this oil. The oil has a deep blue color.

Chamomile Roman - Valuable for soothing the central nervous system and relieving cramps spasms and muscle pains. It also has analgesic effects which may be used for wounds. In humans this has traditionally been used for teething. **Horse** - The strong analgesic properties relieve dull muscular aches and stubborn spasms. It can also relieve overworked and inflamed muscles. Can be used as a wash to relieve the pain of inflames wounds. Good for calming difficult and unruly horses. Good for unmanageable mares when they cycle.

Cinnamon Leaf - Use the leaf not the bark as the leaf is gentler. Excellent digestive tonic and good for flatulent dogs and is a powerful anti-microbial.

Citronella - Well known insect repeller.

Clary Sage - Sedates the central nervous system, good for calming blends. **Horse** - Has a strong regenerative power where hair loss is involved. Useful on puffy joints caused by long periods of standing. Any swelling in the kidney area caused by strenuous work or sluggish kidney function. Calms underlying tension and soothes anxiety. Useful for a mare having trouble conceiving or nervous of the stallion. Don't use during pregnancy.

Coriander Seed - A toning balancing and strengthening oil that promotes and supports the digestion. It is also a circulatory stimulant and thus a good addition to blends for sore joints, muscles or arthritis.

Eucalyptus Radiata - A well-known remedy for congestion of the respiratory system. The oil has anti-viral, anti-inflammatory and expectorant effects. Can be a flea repellant. Antidotes Homoeopathic remedies. **Horse** - Eases muscular aches and pains caused by over exertion, relieves rheumatic and nerve pains. The anti-viral action is good for respiratory infections and it also soothes the inflammation and reduces excess mucous. Heals sores prone to pus formation. Can be irritating to sensitive skin.

Frankincense - Used to strengthen a weakened immune system and is a good choice for any blend for a sick or elderly animal that needs a systemic boost. Can be used for skin aliments due to its anti-inflammatory and anti-bacterial qualities. Horse - Eases shortness of breath and helps any respiratory problem. Rejuvenating especially for those recovering from a serious injury, tonic for the aging and can be used as a pick me up. Good for stubborn hard to heal wounds. Has the ability to dispel fear and anxiety. Don't use during pregnancy.

Geranium - Has tonic and strong anti-fungal actions, suitable in the use of prevention and treatment of fungal ear infections. Also can be used in tick repellant formulas. **Horse** - Gentle analgesic, has diuretic properties and a tonic action on the liver and kidneys. Balance hormones and emotions so is good for erratic mood swings.

Ginger - Good for the digestive and circulatory systems. Used for motion sickness, sprains, strains and arthritis. **Horse** - Good for conditions caused by cold and dampness. Stimulates circulation to cold joints and is analgesic relieving arthritic and rheumatic pain, muscle spasms and sprains. Is a appetite stimulant and can relieve travel sickness. Careful on sensitive skins.

Grapefruit - Used for calming, deodorizing and also repelling insects particularly fleas. Has a tonic effect on skin, hair and tissues. Useful for animals with imbalanced sebum production. **Horse** - Gentle effective lymphatic stimulant that nourishes cells while removing toxins. Tonic to the liver. Careful on sensitive skins.

Helichrysum - Actions - Analgesic, anti-inflammatory, regenerative, good for the skin.

Hyssop Decumbens - Different from the normal hyssop. This one is a antiviral and antibacterial and anti-depressant. The oil is also nontoxic and irritating.

Juniper Berry - Stimulating to the circulatory system and good for use in blends used for arthritis and pain. Helpful for balancing oily skin and for acne, eczema and hair loss. **Horse** - Helps stimulate kidney function and this in turn helps to remove metabolic wastes. Don't use during pregnancy.

Labdunum - This oil is antibacterial and astringent. Used for wounds.

Lavender - Antibacterial, antipruritic (anti-itch), powerful regenerative properties. The oil acts as a sedative on the central nervous system. **Horse** - Is cell regenerating and hastens the healing process. Sedates and soothes any wound or emotion. Helps to dispel gas and eases muscle tightness.

Lemon - Calming, strong antibacterial, deodorizer. **Horse** - Stimulates the body to excrete toxins and wastes via the skin, gently astringent and encourages the movement and release of excess toxins. Supports the liver and kidneys. In the cold season gently addresses runny watery respiratory problems and boosts the immune system. For older horses it can be added to rheumatic blends.

Lemon Grass - Antiviral and has a calming effect. **Horse** - Relieves pain in aching muscles and makes the muscles supple. Careful on sensitive skin and around wounds.

Mandarin Green - Good for calming fear, anxiety or stress. **Horse** - Nourishes the peripheral circulation feeding any extremity that suffers from poor circulation. Helps with muscle spasms.

Marjoram - Calming, spasmolytic, strong antibacterial, bacterial infections, wound care and insect repelling.
Meant to be good for calming over amorous male dogs. **Horse** - Warms cold aching joints, relieves muscle spasms and draws bruising to the surface. Helps with the aches and pain of arthritis and swollen joints in old horses. Can help with travel sickness.

Myrrh - Anti-inflammatory, anti-viral, good for puppy teething, treating irritated or inflamed skin conditions or for adding to immune boosting blends. Good for repelling ticks. **Horse** - Its antiseptic action is useful for deep seated respiratory conditions when inhaled. Can be used in a compress to treat boils, chapped or weeping skin conditions and fungal conditions like ringworm. Has a stimulating toning action on the mares reproductive system. Use only short term and not during pregnancy.

Neroli - Calming, stress reduction, anxiety, used for blend for female dogs in labor to ease pain and stress.

Niaouli - Anti histamine, antibacterial, good for allergies manifesting on the skin as well as first aid. Use for cleaning and for preventing ear infections in dogs.

Nutmeg - Canine flatulence, reduces gas production and aids in indigestion and nausea. Stimulating to the circulatory system.

Sweet Orange - Calming, deodorizing, flea repellant, may help in excess sebum production of the skin.

Palmarosa - Antibacterial, antiviral. **Horse** - Helpful when the body is over heated, encourages cellular regeneration and aid hydration by encouraging the flow of fluids throughout the body. Good for stiff joints and aching back.

Patchouli - Gentle circulatory stimulant for the skin and coat and also acts as a insect repellant. **Horse** - Tissue regenerator that aids in the healing of wounds, may address old scar tissue if applied regularly. Used for treating sores that contain heat a compress will cool the wound and help heal. Helps the skin regain its elasticity. Has diuretic properties.

Peppermint - Stimulates circulation, analgesic, sprains, strains, arthritis, repels fleas, flies, mossies', itching, car sickness. **Horse** - Peppermint has a cooling and analgesic action on heated local injuries. Can burn sensitive skins. Antidotes Homoeopathics.

Ravensare - Anti viral and antibacterial. For animals with compromised immune systems or for young dogs that are prone to infections.

Rose - Stabilizing to the central nervous system, has a gentle tonifying effect to the skin good for adding to blends for itchy or irritated skin.

Rosemary - The oil is mucolytic acting as a expectorant and also aids in cell regeneration. May help in promoting and maintaining hair growth.

Horse - Stimulates both the mental and physical body into action, can relieve pain without sedating.

Rosewood - The oil has antiviral and antibacterial properties and ticks are repelled by the scent of it. Good for skin conditions.

Spearmint - Similar actions to peppermint, repels fleas and other insects stimulates circulation to the area it is used.

Spikenarde - Calming and grounding, rejuvenating and regenerating to the skin, good for dogs with skin problems, has a similar range of action as valerian.

Thyme Linalol - Antibacterial, anti-fungal, good for skin problems and not as harsh as thyme.

Thyme Thujanol - Has all the benefits of the above thyme as well as being a immune system stimulant and live detoxifier. Can be used in the prevention of lymes disease applied immediately after a tick bite.

Valerian - Calming and grounding, good for dogs with separation anxiety or who are fearful of loud noises, storms, fireworks or new situations. Good as a tonic for the nervous system.

Vetiver - Used in blends for calming, circulatory

tonic and strengthens the immune system. **Horse** - Used to treat aches and pains and is a tonic for most body systems. Used for debilitated and distressed horses.

Ylang Ylang - Deeply calming, used in fatigue blends. **Horses** - Commonly used as a aphrodisiac, has an affinity for the adrenal glands.

Vitamin C

Vitamin C is the primary antioxidant in the lungs and a powerful antihistamine without side effects. Low vitamin C dramatically increases histamine levels which put you at greater risks for inflammation responses in the body. Always give a high dose of Vitamin C to animals before any operation where they require a anesthetic for the reasons mentioned above as they will recover faster and better from the anesthetic and maybe the inflammation from the surgical incisions will be toned down a bit.

Vitamin C is needed by the immune system and is necessary for healing and the prevention of infections along with being a potent antioxidant with anti-bacterial and antiviral actions. It is also essential for the utilization of the essential amino acids lysine (anti-viral) and proline. Another point to consider is that stress depletes the body's supply of Vitamin C so this may be another factor in the cause of many diseases. Vit C is essential for the formation of collagen tissue which is vital in tendons and cartilage so always consider this in muscle and back injuries and especially trauma injuries.

Sodium Ascorbate is good for use on animals as it is virtually tasteless when added to the animal's food and does not curdle milk. This can be used in high doses when needed for example dose till the bowels become loose then back the dose off. For severe situations you can use a injectable Vitamin C, in Australia we use Troys Injectable Vit C which we get from the Agricultural Stock Feed Shops or Co Ops. Use a large gauge needle with this as some animals have rather thick hides and the liquid solution is also fairly thick.

Think of using Vitamin C in all operations and all acute diseases. It is a good last resort to think of before the rifle especially in the deadly acute diseases where as a last resort you would use the injectable form in a intramuscular injection, this can also be a good gauge as to what may happen as these injections hurt like hell so if the animal turns around and gives you a filthy look then there is a good chance that they may live and if they do not seem to notice the injection well the chances don't look too good. So remember always keep a bottle of Injectable C in the fridge for emergencies.

Good Herb Sources Of Vitamin C

Alfalfa, Burdock, Catnip, Cayenne, Chickweed, Dandelion, Hawthorn, Garlic, Horseradish, Kelp, Parsley, Plantain, Papaya, Raspberry, Rosehips, Shepherds Purse, Yellow Dock.

Notes

Notes

Notes

Notes

Notes

Notes

Notes

www.ingramcontent.com/pod-product-compliance
Lightning Source LLC
Chambersburg PA
CBHW051500170526
45166CB00001B/326